JUST ENOUGH TO BE GREAT IN YOUR DENTAL PROFESSION

Just Enough to be Great in your Dental Profession

Processes and Procedures for Success

Kevin Coughlin DMD

ISBN: 1508705933
ISBN 13: 9781508705932
Library of Congress Control Number: 2015903720
CreateSpace Independent Publishing Platform
North Charleston, South Carolina

I would like to dedicate this study guide to a group of individuals who have helped and supported me since 1983 in the development of one of the best dental organizations anywhere. Calling these individuals "employees" does not do them justice. Every day, this team provides the highest level of service and care in an unending pursuit to help our most important asset: our patient base. This group of dedicated individuals, in most instances, receives very little fanfare or acknowledgment. Yet the team is constantly helping and continuing to develop processes and procedures that consistently provide growth, expansion, and success for our dental company, Baystate Dental. My goal is not to make us specialists but to provide great general dentistry by creating a study guide of best business and clinical practices. I thank you all so very much!

Tracey Andrew, Nicole Antaya, Tamara Arbuzov, Marcie Aubin, Lesia Avraamova, Jillian Barnard, Nadezhda Belyshev, Christine Benvenuto, Erin Bishop, Marilee Boothe, Debra Boucher, Marcie Brunelle, Catherine Byrne, Paul Byrne, Beth Castaldo, Donna ChinSee, Jean Clouse, Laura Cortes, Karen Coughlin, Joyce Coughlin, Ralph Coughlin, Susan Crochetiere, Debbie Davis, Ivana De Los Santos, Kristin Desilets, Richard Drummond, Jessica Drzewianowski, Julie Eldridge, Natalie Figaro, Mary Garvey, Laura Girard, Nicole Gloster, Ashley Greco, Roberta Guthrie, Becky Guyette, Amy Guyon, Jonathan Haluch, Stacy Haluch, Michelle Hartnett, Debra Hilton, Monika Jagodzinska, Sara Jambard, Juan Jimenez, Theresa Kaplan, Mary Kelly, Anna Kutergin, Catherine LaFountain, Billie Lahr, Victoria Laughney, Sonja Lavigne, Suzanne Leh, Amber Leneau, Rachael Letourneau, Irina Leyderer, Nicole Lipp, Gundi Lobo, Jessica Lopez, Joan Luchini, Diana Luong, Patricia Marszalek, Richard Marszalek, Vicki Martin, Mariam Martinez, Wilfredo Martinez, Scott Massey, Nelya Mecher, Judith Miarecki, Nicole Miner, Heather Mulrooney, Julie Murphy, Jovan Newson, Emily Nicodemi, Kaitlyn O'Connell, Janice O'Connell, Linda O'Leary, Jessie Oliveira, Bridget O'Neill, Ovysdioel Ortiz, Roberto Ortiz, Carolyn Ostrowski, Marina Panchenko, Carly Phillips, Melissa Pires, Patricia Porter, Cindy Rivera, Kelly Rivera, Cara Roberge, Erin Rosario, Wanda Ruiz, Megan Samson, Kayla Sanchez, Amber Sanders, Aleida Santos, Ann Marie Santos, Cheryl Schnepp, Babak Seihoun, Katherine Shelton, Karen Shidell, Janie Sieracki, Diane Silva, Patricia Silva, Bernadette Sole, Kathleen St. Germain, Jessica Tabb, Sara Jean Taylor, Martha Thompson, Alisa Torres, Carmen Torres, Natalie, Torres, Amy Turcotte, Vilandria Turney, Amanda Vallone, Melissa Vandermyn, Beth Vanlderstine, Latresse Waldon, Andrea Walsh, Jennah Whitcomb, Larendalys Wilson, Jodi Woodbury and Monique Worm

A special thanks to Ms. Carmen Torres; your battle is our battle. We love you and thank you for everything…

CONTENTS

INTRODUCTION

To me, T.E.A.M. means "together employees achieve mastership." Since 1983, I, along with the help of many others, have created the best dental organization possible. During this time, I have made numerous mistakes because I lacked the experience, knowledge, training, and expertise to achieve this goal. My assumption is that I am not unique. I surmise that other dental organizations, large and small, have had very similar problems. I have created a training manual that gets to the heart of the matter and that can be used as a guide by dentists and their staff to create a better environment, one that is more efficient and effective at creating the highest level of care and service not only for our patient base but for our teams. The best way to achieve this goal is to examine and evaluate every part of your dental practice and then to design, review, and develop appropriate processes and procedures to achieve those goals.

1. Developing Your Team

Consider training, education, attitude, and money as the building blocks for creating your team. I believe individuals over the age of thirty who want and need employment will be your best starting point in developing your team. I came to this conclusion after evaluating thousands of employees across three decades. I have decided that commitment, loyalty, trust, and desire are the hallmarks in developing a highly trained and motivated team. This is not to imply that younger employees cannot be a wonderful asset. However, the long-term success of holding on to younger employees, considering the changes that they go through during their development, makes it very difficult for them to stay employed with your organization for a long period of time.

Other traits also are important in the evaluation and construction of your team. Some characteristics to consider are whether potential employees are married, single, or have a history involving a long-term relationship. I bring this up because a successful team is very similar to a successful relationship, in that it requires maturity, devotion, loyalty, forgiveness, and the ability to work through problems and come to successful, stable outcomes. Characteristics such as employees' children and the ages of those children create another set of potential issues. The team member with young children, in most cases, will always have to put his or her children before your business; this can create anxiety, stress, and problems.

Keep in mind that although many of my thoughts and recommendations will be successful for any business, my personal area of expertise is in the dental field. In most cases, the average dental office will have fewer than ten employees. In such small-office situations, the depth and number of employees make it more difficult for the owner to meet his or her staff's wants and needs while also providing exceptional care and service to his or her patients. In small-group organizations, when an individual has to leave early due to family commitments, illness, and so forth, it is difficult to maintain a high level of care and service in your organization. This can, and in most cases will, become an issue.

The next set of characteristics I look for in developing an extraordinary team is an individual's background in sales and marketing combined with business knowledge. This person also should be energetic, caring, and a team player. In addition to those characteristics, a clinical background in the field of dentistry is an extraordinary advantage but not a necessity. If forced to make a decision between someone who is knowledgeable and someone who has great sales and management skills, I would always pick the latter. Clinical skills can more easily be taught; teaching management and sales are much more difficult.

I suggest that you build your team around individuals with a background and knowledge of dental assisting and dental hygiene. I would be lying if I said it is easy to find such individuals; in fact, it is extremely difficult. In some cases, it may appear impossible, but it can be done. There is an old adage in business that for every $10,000 you pay a staff member, it takes you one month to find that right individual. What that means is that if you're going to pay someone $50,000 a year on average, it will take you five months to find that particular individual. I emphasize that no matter how much effort and time are necessary, such precision will be worth it in the long run. It is a critical step in accomplishing your goal of developing the ideal dental business. Not selecting the right individuals when creating your team will result in an enormous cost to you and your organization. This step should not be taken lightly.

I also recommend that in the process of hiring and developing your team you consider your patient base. Whether your community is mostly African American, Hispanic, of European descent, or Caucasian, single, married, young, or old, look for individuals with whom your patient base will be most comfortable. As time goes on, such conditions may evolve to be less important; however, make no mistake about it: individuals are more comfortable around similar individuals. That said, I also think some diversity in your team can create untapped business opportunities for your organization. You will find that as your staff becomes more diversified so will your patient base, provided you follow proper procedures and processes. Remember that your staff should be one of your greatest sources of referrals; they will send family and friends to your organization.

The processes and procedures of hiring your team should revolve around the following guidelines.

A dental practice with a patient base of roughly two thousand active patients (meaning such patients visit your practice at least once every eighteen months) and

An office space of twenty-five hundred to three thousand square feet, containing four to six dental operatories that can provide a wide range of services, in most cases requires the following:

- Three full-time individuals at your front-desk area
- One to two full-time dental hygienists
- Two to three full-time dental assistants

This will provide you with enough depth and overlap to keep your team happy and organized.

In summary, you have selected your team: individuals over the age of thirty who are married (any children are over the age of twelve) and are dedicated, trustworthy, energetic team players with knowledge of sales, business, and dentistry. Ideally, they have been or can be dental assistants.

2. Developing Processes and Procedures

First, I will address the front-desk team member. This, in my opinion, is the most important starting point because he or she is usually the patient's first and last point of contact. The areas that need to be developed are as follows:

- Telephone skills
- Gathering data
- Interpreting the data
- Patient orientation
- Developing and providing information about a comprehensive treatment plan
- Developing and reviewing financial options for the patient to receive care and treatment
- The systems to follow up with those patients who have or have not accepted treatment
- The reports needed to assess the success and progress of your business team
- Review of changes and developments that constantly need to be evaluated in making necessary adjustments accordingly, through daily, biweekly, weekly, or monthly meetings and discussions

Let us first discuss the processes and procedures associated with answering the phone. I suggest the following: "This is Dr. Smith's office. Thank you for calling. How may we help you?" What's important to understand is that you are identifying the office name, you are thanking the individual for selecting your office for care, and, lastly, you are showing your willingness and ability to help the individual with his or her real or perceived problem. Please do not underestimate the power of that simple opening. Your front-desk team should never do the following: "This is Dr. Smith's office. I have to put you on hold." No matter how busy or how stressed, I recommend that your team be able to answer that phone in fewer than four rings. If that is not possible (and many times, it will not be), you must have a system in place that gives your patient a choice. He or she can leave his or her name, phone number, and any questions. You must then let the caller know you will return his or her call within fifteen minutes. Alternatively, the caller has the option to stay on the line and, every thirty seconds, the caller is reminded that he or she has not been forgotten and someone will be with him or her momentarily. If this process takes more than two minutes, the patient on the phone should have the option to be contacted within the next fifteen minutes.

It is critical that your front-desk team understands that in most cases, an individual does not want to listen to a recording, does not want to be kept on hold, and will want his or her questions answered honestly and fairly as soon as possible. This is why the individual answering the phone must be among the strongest members of your team. He or she must possess patience, knowledge, grace under pressure, and the ability to show empathy, along with being efficient and effective in achieving a result. Simply stated, when a patient hangs up the phone, his or her problem either has been resolved or will be resolved within the next fifteen minutes.

For most readers, this may appear to be a very simplistic task. However, I urge you to have a colleague or friend contact your office or for you to attempt phone duty yourself. You will see how demanding, difficult, and often times impossible it is to perform. From their perspectives, your patients think your front-desk attendant has endless amounts of time to answer all their questions, clinical and financial, when in reality your employee will be multi-tasking due to people checking in and checking out at the front desk. Doctors could be asking questions too as he or she tries to handle additional incoming phone calls. In the real world, it is often impossible to provide proper care and service to those individuals waiting at the front desk or on the phone. For those phone conversations that are outside the normal standard call, I recommend, simply, straightforwardly, and honestly saying, "Mr. or Ms. Smith, it is important that I resolve this issue. Please allow me to get back to you later on today. Is there a time or number that is best for me to reach you?"

For those individuals standing at the front desk, I recommend that you have them simply take a seat in your consultation room, provided you have one. If you do not, I recommend they take a seat in your reception room until you can address their issues.

Some desirable qualities of individuals answering the phone are a clear, comforting voice and an ability to show sincerity and concern.

As I continue to discuss incoming phone calls, understand that the majority will be as follows:

- To make an appointment
- To cancel an appointment
- To change an appointment time or date
- To ask about services that are provided
- To ask about insurance coverage and/or remaining benefits
- To inquire about financial issues
- To complain about previous care and/or treatment

To grasp fully the enormous difficulties of phone duty, please consider the litany of other incoming calls, all of which are important in projecting the image of your business and have nothing directly to do with your dental practice. Examples of these would be husbands, wives, boyfriends, or girlfriends wanting to speak to the doctor or other employees; insurance companies inquiring about claims and information; pharmacies calling about prescriptions; outside vendors requesting conversations with doctors and staff; and attorneys and accountants, along with banks, looking to speak to the owner or owners regarding the operation's day-to-day business decisions. Although on the surface such calls do not relate directly to patient care, how they are handled is nonetheless a reflection on you, your business, and your team. The same importance and emphasis should be placed on these calls as on any other call. This type of phone call, in my opinion, should be dealt with during nontreatment times, such as before the day starts, during breaks, during lunch, at the end of the day, or during time off. Every successful phone conversation should lead to a positive feeling about you and your organization.

THE PHONE CONVERSATION ASSOCIATED WITH MAKING AN APPOINTMENT

After answering the phone properly, you must first establish the following.

- What is the patient's chief complaint?
- Is this patient a new or existing patient?

Remember, good service in almost all cases will trump good care. It should be obvious that the goal is to provide not just excellent service but also excellent care. When you establish the nature of the patient's chief complaint, it shows that you and your team care. If there is no chief complaint and the patient is an existing patient, establishing the time and location of an appointment and attempting to meet your patients' needs and goals within limitations become paramount.

It is my experience that the majority of your patients will want either early morning, lunch time, evening, or weekend appointments. If your organization does not offer those options, I strongly recommend that you create such options for your patients if you are truly serious about establishing outstanding care and service.

For the patient who has a chief complaint, the art is determining the level of concern that the patient has in regard to that complaint. Understand that from the clinical side, many times we, as dental professionals, will not consider the patient's chief complaint to be serious. Trust me, for an individual to call your dental office, he or she feels his or her complaint is very serious. I suggest that after establishing the patient's chief complaint, you try to quantify his or her level of concern by asking, "Mr. or Ms. Smith, on a pain scale from zero to ten, with ten being the worst pain and zero being no pain at all, what would you consider your pain level to be?" After the level of pain is established, I recommend that you follow up by asking, "Is this problem top, bottom, right, left, front, or back?" The location of the problem or problems provides important information. For example, if it is a front tooth, most patients will consider it a higher priority than a back tooth because it will show. Back teeth are usually more difficult to provide root-canal therapy or perform extractions on compared to front teeth. Lower teeth are more difficult to provide local anesthesia than upper teeth. Establishing location helps the front-desk coordinator determine the amount of time needed for an appointment and, perhaps, the seriousness of the problem.

After the chief complaint is established, I recommend focusing on the duration of the problem. "Mr. or Ms. Smith, how long has this problem been bothering you? Mr. or Ms. Smith, is this something that you want us to address today or over the next few days? Thank you so much for calling us. I know we will be able to resolve your problem." The responses to the above questions create a profile for Mr. or Ms. Smith. If you think about it, someone who states he or she has a pain level of ten and duration of more than a few days has clearly been holding off on care and treatment due to fear, finances, or a combination of both. Keep in mind that each patient's perception of his or her problem depends on a combination of factors. Extremely busy individuals will often put off care and treatment as long as possible because it's an inconvenience to his or her schedule; he or she simply does not have the time to receive care. Others have nothing but time but lack the financial resources to obtain care. Still others are somewhere in the middle, wise enough to understand they require care and treatment but hope their issues will resolve on their own.

In all cases, I recommend you offer a patient either the option to come in immediately or sometime that day. This is an important concept to understand. I am well aware that you may not be able to accommodate Mr. or Ms. Smith on that particular day. However, my experience tells me that most people are just interested in knowing whether they can be seen that day, but they may not actually be willing to come in for their appointment. The important point is that they are offered the opportunity to come in to have their issue or chief complaint evaluated. Understand that as a patient coordinator or team member, getting someone in is different than necessarily getting something done. In the first case, having someone come in for evaluation of his or her chief complaint, taking a radiograph, and coming up with the diagnosis, treatment plan, and perhaps prescriptions are all that will be needed. Actual care can be done on another day. If the chief complaint is severe, in most cases a properly well-trained staff should be able to resolve the problem by opening the tooth and allowing for drainage in the case of an abscess, whether the abscess is tooth or tissue in nature. Your team should be able to extract the tooth or provide some type of temporary or long-lasting restoration. For offices that avoid specialty care, a prescription and referral often are all that is necessary to satisfy that patient's chief complaint.

I am a firm believer that for the general dental practice, the more specialty care that you can deliver the better your overall service and care will be. Although most dentists feel that it's simpler or easier and less stressful to delegate specialty care out to dental specialists, it is my belief that most general dentists should be able to provide over 90 percent of all treatment as long as adequate effort and training are present. The tremendous goodwill that is created in helping Mr. and Ms. Smith beyond the radiograph and referral slip cannot be overstated. In today's environment, high degrees of specialization have created an almost impossible scenario for patients to receive any kind of treatment from start to finish, and the resulting costs in time and inconvenience for your patient base is enormous. The potential loss of revenue and goodwill caused by such practices should be avoided. Remember, the goal of your dental practice should be to create what I refer to as "raving fans," the individuals who support your practice and are so satisfied with your care and service that they cannot help but tell family, friends, and associates.

Developing what I refer to as the BLT—or the "believe, like, and trust" factor—over the phone is critical. In order for your team to accomplish this, its members must determine if a caller is a new patient or an existing patient. If he or she is a new patient, after the chief complaint has been established, I recommend a comment such as, "We have seen many problems like this in the past, and I am quite confident our team will be able to assist you and solve your problem." If the caller is an existing patient, a specific series of steps and procedures should be developed. In this case, you first should know the date of the patient's last visit to your office.

Anyone whose last appointment was over a year ago should be handled differently than a patient who was last seen within the past twelve months. In particular, a patient who has not been to your office for more than twelve months requires updated records and should be treated just like a new patient. This will require evaluation of or new bitewing radiographs, an updated clinical exam, and a hygiene appointment.

To get deeper into the discussion of this matter, you should examine why the patient has not visited in more than twelve months. Is it simply because your processes, procedures, or recall are poor, or is it that the patient has refused to commit to treatment? In most cases, the issues are fear, finances, or time. It is important to assess whether it is fear, finances, time, or some combination. To avoid lack of care and service in the future, it is important to ascertain the patient's reason for delaying care.

When it comes to fear, I recommend that you offer some type of sedation option. In general, I strongly recommend that your organization consider oral sedation, inhalation sedation, intravenous sedation, or general anesthesia that can be administered in your office or at an area hospital. Proper training and education in these areas can create an opportunity to grow and expand your patient base.

If the patient's issue is financial, you should evaluate which insurance plans you are accepting and not accepting, as well as whether you would like to participate in plans that you are currently not involved with and their various ramifications in cost, time, and finances to your organization. Evaluating your options—including whether your organization accepts outside financial arrangements such as credit cards, Care Credit, Wells Fargo, and similar financial programs that establish a line of credit to your new and existing patients—will allow you to offer more comprehensive care and treatment to your patient base.

If time is the issue and it prevents your patients from seeking care, you must consider being open early in the morning, during lunch, during evenings, and on weekends if you are serious about exceptional care and service.

Since starting my dental practice in 1983 and averaging over nine hundred new patients a month from my fourteen offices, I can definitely tell you that the number-one reason patients leave their current dentist and seek care somewhere else is because their existing office no longer accepts their dental plan or insurance. The second major reason is that the individual could not get an appointment that was convenient for him or her and his or her family. The third is that the patient was provided with no financial options, meaning the patient feels that he or she would not be able to afford care and service at this particular time. The fourth major reason patients move on is that they are tired of dental offices charging for an exam, consultation, and radiograph and then referring them out while their primary problem or chief complaint was left unresolved or untreated.

My goal is not to create a dentist who never refers, but I do think after four years of college, four years of dental school, and, in most cases, additional training beyond that, the majority of us should be able to do some specialty care. Certain conditions should be resolvable by a general dentist. For example, most dentists should be able to perform the placement of a single implant with appropriate width and height of bone and soft tissue. With even a moderate amount of training and experience, you should be able to surgically place and restore missing teeth with dental implants.

In further discussing the conditions associated with a patient and after determining whether the patient has visited your establishment within the previous twelve months, you should evaluated the patient's insurance situation, the patient's financial and appointment history with the practice, and the number of referrals and family members associated with the patient. Let us first safely assume that given proper office processes and procedures, the loss of a single patient will almost never occur. In almost all cases, when an individual leaves a practice due to dissatisfaction of any type, his or her significant others—husband, wife, partner, children, friends, or some combination—will also be leaving. The costs or opportunity costs associated with the loss of all those individuals are almost impossible to quantify, but I can assure you that they are significant. As you establish the type of patient, you should also be able to evaluate the finances associated with a particular patient. What I mean by this involves a simple, straightforward approach. Coding or evaluating your patient base could entail the following:

- Type I patients generally have no insurance and pay for their care out of pocket.
- Type II patients are generally over the age of sixty-five and, one would assume, no longer responsible for the finances of their children. Their homes in most cases will be paid off, and, after years of putting off care and treatment for themselves to provide for their family, they are in a position to start taking care of their needs.
- Type III patients are those individuals who have an insurance plan but that insurance plan allows the dental organization to balance the bill.
- Type IV patients are those on some type of government-assistance plan due to significant financial restraints.
- Type V patients are individuals with a type of insurance plan in which the dental organization signs a contract agreeing to accept a reduced fee but that in many cases will not allow you to balance bill to your ordinary and customary fees.

Although these categories can produce many subcategories, quantifying these five particular types will enable the front-desk coordinator to maximize the potential dollars that can be produced and expected to be collected.

The next part of the patient profile is a financial profile based on processes and procedures: does the patient have a history of paying bills in full or within thirty days? A soft credit check can be performed to determine whether the patient is a high or low risk to internal financial arrangements or such external financial arrangements as those established by Care Credit or Wells Fargo. Each office will have its particular sets of wants and needs based on how its organization is set up.

I personally feel that the best, most cost-effective group of patients to treat from a business standpoint is those who fall into the types I and II categories and who have been preapproved by a soft credit check. Discussing patients' financial needs and wants based on their insurance as well as issues such as what will be approved and not approved, what is within and outside the plan, and what treatment is and is not covered takes an enormous amount of time, energy, and effort from your staff. The ability to simply quote a fee and not have to discuss insurance issues is a tremendous boon to your organization, and I would strongly suggest you try to cultivate those individuals in your practice.

After the front-desk coordinator establishes the patient type and his or her financial situation, the next logical hurdle is scheduling issues. An example might be an individual with a swollen face, a pain level eight out of ten, severe discomfort, the duration of the problem is more than a week, or lack of financial means. In this case, it simply makes no sense to schedule a ninety-minute appointment for root-canal buildup and a crown. The well-trained front-desk coordinator should be able to determine that this situation calls for either an exam and radiograph with a prescription or an extraction, and in either case a ninety-minute appointment would be an extremely inefficient use of time, for both your office and your patient. In collecting and assessing the data and information, a well-trained front-desk coordinator should be able to ascertain, based on the potential dollars produced, whether it makes sense to tie up prime time in the schedule—generally early morning, lunch hour, and evening and weekend appointments—or to look for scheduling during low or nonproducing appointment times. These include side-booked appointments or appointments in the 9:00 a.m.–11:00 a.m. or 2:00 p.m.–4:00 p.m. time frames. I recommend that with this group of patients, you guide them toward nonprime time slots.

FOR CALLS REGARDING CANCELING OR CHANGING A PATIENT'S APPOINTMENT

You should first establish if there is any way this can be avoided. I recommend that you consider the distinctions of broken appointments versus last-minute cancelations and have them coded into your software system.

A patient who has a broken appointment (BA) is someone who did not show for an appointment and neglected to give the front-desk coordinator at least forty-eight hours' notice. A patient with a last-minute cancelation (LMC) is someone who had the courtesy and respect at least to inform you that something came up and he or she needs to reschedule. These are two distinct types of patients, and it is important that your front-desk coordinator make the distinction. The individual who does not provide at least forty-eight hours' notice will have the tendency to forget not just about his or her dental care but about other appointments as well. These patients are generally more concerned with what is important to them rather than what is important to you and your organization. Please do not take this the wrong way: this does not to mean that they are good or bad people; it simply means that dental care and dental health are not high priorities for them. This is in contrast to the majority of cases of patients with a last-minute cancelation. In general such patients will appreciate others people's time and expertise but, for a variety of reasons, are unable to keep an appointment. I suggest that in your processes and procedures you code the missing appointments as either a BA for broken appointment or LMC for last-minute cancelation. When the phone rings in your office, the front-desk coordinator should be able to tell immediately whether the calling patient has a history of missed appointments and, if so, whether those appointments were broken appointments or last-minute cancelations.

FOR CALLS TO INQUIRE ABOUT PROCEDURES, CARE, AND SERVICE

I cannot emphasize how critical it is to have a clinically trained individual answering such calls. Imagine a patient who is interested in implants, extractions, and upper or lower fixed or removable prostheses and has concerns and questions about whether the office provides those services and care. How would you feel, as an existing patient or a potential new patient, if the front-desk coordinator says, "I am so sorry; I cannot answer those questions. I am not sure whether we provide that level of care and service."

I advocate that the front-desk coordinator be able to answer the full array of the lay public's questions, including such subjects as:

- Radiographs (how and when they are performed)
- Extractions (what can be expected regarding postoperative discomfort, how long they take, and how much they cost)
- Implants (why we recommend them, when they should be recommended, and how much they cost)
- Periodontal or gum infections and periodontal care (what is entailed, the potential pain, and how much it costs)
- Headaches, jaw pain, limited range of motion, or simply TMJ treatment (when is treatment performed, what is involved, and how much it costs)

The list can go on, but in general, speaking strictly from a business and sales perspective, I have emphasized over the entire course of my career that the front-desk coordinator has to have knowledge and information about all clinical procedures the office provides. The first and perhaps most important issue when it comes to your front-desk coordinator is skill in getting patients into the office for the correct amount of time and the appropriate slot in your appointment schedule. The front-desk coordinator is an educator and sales person—make no mistake about it. Secondly, a front-desk coordinator must have the skills of a clinician in order to evaluate the seriousness of problems and assess the steps and the time necessary to resolve them. As a rule, I train all front-desk coordinators to respond to almost any patient condition by telling the caller that he or she can come immediately to our office for evaluation. The exception is when the front-desk coordinator feels that a true or potentially life-threatening emergency is apparent. In those cases, the patient should immediately go to the emergency room. Examples might be if a patient says he or she is having difficulty swallowing or speaking; in that case, the obvious fear is a potential airway obstruction. Severe swelling, rash, hives, and a potentially serious allergic reaction could be imminent, and, again, such patients should be immediately seen at the ER. Another potential exception might be uncontrolled bleeding when pressure on the wound for eight to ten minutes does not stop the bleeding.

In almost all other circumstances, you should request patients to come in as soon as possible for evaluation. The front-desk coordinator must fully understand that a patient arriving at the office for an appointment does not necessarily mean he or she will be receiving treatment; it may simply mean an evaluation, discussion, and another appointment in the future based on clinical circumstances and the type of patient. It may be difficult to find skilled front-desk coordinators with such knowledge, which is why having systems in place to provide training and education is absolutely necessary.

I recommend that you develop a webpage that addresses all the areas of dentistry: orthodontics, periodontics, endodontic, pediatrics, oral surgery, radiology, pathology, cosmetics, fixed and removable prosthodontics, implantology, sedation, and TMJ. This will allow your front-desk coordinator, especially in times of confusion, hectic schedules, or lack of knowledge, to refer patients to your website to have their questions answered. I also recommend software programs for your organization, not only to educate your patient base but your staff as well. Two excellent programs available are CAESY Cloud and Consult-PRO. Both provide oral and digital images and explanations of almost every clinical dental situation you can imagine.

FOR CALLS REGARDING INSURANCE

The caller may ask whether a certain procedure is covered and details about remaining benefits that are available on his or her plan. In almost all dental software programs, you should be able to evaluate quickly and efficiently the remaining benefits on an individual or family's plan. In most cases, dental insurance coverage will not pay more than $500, $750, $1,000, $1,500, or $2,000 in a calendar year. In most cases, dental plans are divided into type one, two, and three coverage. Type one involves exams, radiographs, and preventive care. Type two generally involves restorations. Type three involves tooth replacement. Most type one dental coverage pays between 50 percent and 100 percent. Most type two plans cover between 50 percent and 80 percent. In most cases, dental insurance will pay 0 percent to 50 percent of tooth replacement, provided it is not a preexisting condition of less than twelve months.

These are very general terms. Based on your state and the types of dental insurance plans you accept, you should establish data within your software to be able to ascertain such information quickly and efficiently.

Patients also commonly ask, "Do you accept my plan?" The front-desk coordinator must understand that in all cases he or she will need the patient's name, insurance ID number, and type of plan. I cannot emphasize enough the difficulty involved here. While the patient may say that he or she has Delta Dental, CIGNA, MetLife, Aetna, or some other type of insurance, he or she often will not specifically know or have an insurance card or other information to provide the front-desk coordinator with accurate information. Companies like Delta Dental, for example, may have over fifty different plans that are all called "Delta Dental" and vary in coverage.

FOR CALLS INQUIRING ABOUT FINANCIAL OPTIONS OR QUESTIONS REGARDING A PATIENT'S EXISTING BILLS

In such cases, conversations might go as follows. The patient asks the front-desk coordinator why he or she received a bill or statement when his or her insurance company is responsible for paying. These are delicate situations. The majority of US citizens are employees and do not realize that they actually are responsible for the bill and that their insurance company represents them, not the dental business. I recommend that the front-desk coordinator listen to the entire question before interrupting or speaking to the patient. The problem can be resolved by simply telling Mr. or Ms. Smith that the reason he or she is receiving a statement is that his or her insurance company has not completely processed the claim. Until the claim is processed, the total bill is still outstanding.

In reality, a portion has been paid by the patient and a portion has been paid by the insurance company. Your front-desk coordinator should attempt to explain that the dentist's office has supplied the care and treatment and has been responsible for the overhead, supplies, and expertise, but it is still waiting to be paid by you (the patient), by the patient's insurance company, or both. When this situation occurs, I can assure you that procedures and processes have not been followed or have never been put in place. In such instances, the front-desk coordinator would be wise simply to let the patient know that the office will follow up with the insurance company to make sure that everything has been submitted and received correctly.

Although it seems obvious to someone who has been in business—particularly in the medical or dental fields—for some time, errors do occur. Such errors can be due to the dental office submitting inaccurate information or omitting certain information, causing the insurance company to process the claim incompletely or incorrectly. Another source of errors entails the insurance company making a mistake in processing the claim. In some cases, the patient has actually provided the dental office with inaccurate information, such as an incorrect address, inaccurate date of birth or Social Security number, and the list goes on. The well-trained front-desk coordinator must be able to respond to each situation and make the appropriate corrections. It is very important that you follow up with your patient's wishes and assure him or her that if a problem occurred, it has been corrected.

FOR CALLS INQUIRING ABOUT THE COSTS OR CHARGES

I urge the front-desk coordinator to consider providing the patient with a price range from lowest to highest instead of quoting an exact fee for a particular procedure. Many patients will simply ask why there is a range, and they want to know the exact fee. In such cases, I recommend explaining that you are not the dentist and that a variety of materials, techniques, and procedures are available to accomplish similar goals. Depending on the clinical situation, the fees can vary considerably. For the patient who presses the front-desk coordinator for an exact fee, I recommend you quote the highest fee in the range and then say it may be lower once the doctor has completed the exam, diagnosis, and treatment plan. In my experience, patients almost never complain about charges lower than a quote. However, we receive complaints almost on a daily basis that a quoted fee has been changed to a higher fee. Take note: always quote the highest fee and then either provide services and care to that fee or provide the care and treatment at the lower fee.

FOR CALLERS WHO COMPLAIN ABOUT CARE OR SERVICE

In most cases, the problems will be among the following.

- A temporary crown has fallen off.
- A tooth that was just filled is sensitive to temperature.
- I just had my teeth cleaned, and my gums and teeth are very sore.
- I just spent a lot of money having a crown inserted, and when I bite down, that is the only thing that touches.
- I just had a crown inserted, and I cannot floss between my teeth.
- I just had an extraction done, and I cannot stand the pain—it seems to be getting worse.
- My child is going through orthodontic care, and a wire is cutting into his or her lip or cheek.
- I just received a denture or a partial denture, and it is hurting me and feels loose.

The list of potential problems is almost never-ending; however, these have proven to be patients' most common complaints. I recommend that you allow patients to vent their frustration and explain the complaints without interruption, no matter how busy you are. On those very rare occasions when you have no other options, I strongly recommend you inform the patient that you are sincerely concerned about the problem, but you are not the dentist. You will let the dentist know as soon as possible, and the dentist will follow up within the hour.

I cannot emphasize enough the importance of making sure, no matter how minor you perceive a patient's problem to be, that it be followed up either by the front-desk coordinator or the dentist. Certain specific responses may help relieve patients of their frustrations and dissatisfactions.

In the example of the loose temporary crown that is completely out, you should consider explaining that dentists use a very semipermeable type of cement, since we know we have to remove the temporary crown in the very near future to try in your final restoration.

When the patient complains that a tooth that was just filled is sensitive, determine the sensitivity on the pain scale (zero to ten) and if the problem seems to be improving, staying the same, or getting worse. In these cases, I strongly recommend that you offer the patient a chance to be seen in the office within the next twenty-four hours. I also recommend that you emphasize that new restorations or fillings in many cases will be in close proximity to the nerve in the tooth, the patient's signs and symptoms are normal, and the issues should resolve on their own without any intervention within seven to ten days.

If the situation does not seem to be typical, then reassure the patient that either a temporary restoration, called an IRM, or immediate restorative material may be placed in the tooth to attempt to calm the nerves down. Such restoration will remain in the patient's mouth for six to twelve weeks and then be removed and replaced with a more permanent type of restoration. In the case of swelling, significant discomfort (greater than six out of ten on the pain scale), and symptoms that worsen over time along with the inability to close down on the tooth, you may recommend an evaluation to determine whether root-canal therapy will be necessary.

When a patient complains that after a hygiene appointment, tissues surrounding the gums are very sore and sensitive, I suggest you remind the patient to use warm salt rinses—one tablespoon of salt in a glass of eight ounces of warm water—and rinse for twenty to forty seconds. I also recommend you inform the patient that many times the hygiene staff has had to remove material below the gum tissue around the tooth, and often that causes some short-term soreness but provides excellent long-term results in removing the inflammatory products that cause dental disease and infection.

When a patient explains that a wire from orthodontic treatment is cutting his or her cheek, I recommend you inform the patient that as the teeth move or drift, shifting occurs for orthodontic purposes. Often the wire needs to be trimmed, but it should not create an issue in the long term.

FOR CALLS WHERE THE PATIENT IS UPSET AND ANGRY

These calls must be taken to heart and addressed immediately. If the true goal is to provide exceptional care and service, the upset or dissatisfied patient must be taken care of efficiently and effectively, and the situation must be followed up on to make sure that patient is satisfied.

3. Initial Contact

Some commonly accepted approaches along with processes and procedures will work well during initial patient contact. I feel it is always professional to address your patient by his or her proper title, such as doctor, attorney, mister, or Ms. If you are not sure of the pronunciation of his or her name, just ask. "Mr. or Ms.—Could you please help me? How do I pronounce your name? Thank you."

I suggest that in most cases some type of inoffensive touch such as a handshake will break the ice. However, be aware that in some religions the handshake may be deemed inappropriate so use common sense.

You can learn a lot about people during the initial contact, and the following will help provide some insight into what to look for. Let us start with body language. Nervous and apprehensive types of patients in many cases will have poor eye contact, are very fidgety and nervous, be embarrassed or ashamed of the condition of their dental health, and will not smile. As the healthcare provider, you should be open, calm, relaxed, and confident and in control. You must avoid being overbearing or a know-it-all. Listen more than speak. Show concern about your patient's problems. Let him or her know you can help and that he or she has made the correct choice in seeking out your care and service.

As a doctor, you should notice the patient's complexion.

Is his or her skin warm or cold to the touch?
Is he or she neat or disheveled?
Is he or she in good shape or overweight?
Does it appear that he or she is concerned with his or her appearance?
How does he or she stand and walk?
Is his or her posture good or poor?
Look at his or her hands and nail beds for color and appearance.
Are his or her eyes clear or cloudy?

You should be able to establish to some degree your patient's personality type: is he or she dominant, inspiring, cautious, sensitive? Understanding these personality traits will help you relate quicker and better with your patient.

Please do not underestimate this information. Patients make decisions emotionally; many times, they will make up their mind in a few minutes whether they will want you to care for and treat them and their family.

One of the biggest mistakes I see is the doctor who immediately starts asking about the patient's medical history and chief complaint. I strongly suggest you start by asking your patient what he or she would like to see accomplished on today's visit, what his or her main concern is, and what he or she did not like about his or her previous dental experiences. In most cases, a dentist will be standing up while his or her patient is sitting in a dental chair. I suggest that you also consider sitting so you are eye-to-eye with your patient. You should be upbeat, smile, and say, "Thank you for allowing me to provide your dental care. I look forward to getting to know you better."

I know it is not always practical, but if it is at all possible, go to the reception room to greet your patient. This simple act will go a long way. The quicker your patient likes, believes, and trusts you, the better off you will both be. This is probably the best information I can provide to the new or seasoned practitioner.

4. New Patient Orientation

I RECOMMEND PATIENT ORIENTATION for individuals who have been out of your office for two years or more or who are new patients to your practice. It should take place in a private room containing educational models and software to help educate patients, as well as marketing materials and information about the doctors in the practice. The objective of the orientation is to establish information about a patient, but it also helps that individual develop a belief in, trust of, and good feelings toward the practice and the staff. The orientation should take on a logical sequence of events. It should always start with "thank you for allowing us to provide your dental care" and a review of the patient's chief complaint. You should reassure the patient that you will be able to solve his or her particular problem and that you have dealt with such issues in the past. After the chief complaint has been discussed, you should review with the patient how long it has been since the last dental appointment, any reasons for the delay in treatment, and reason for not revisiting his or her previous dentist. These issues are very important and can provide enormous information to the front-desk coordinator and doctor.

In most cases, delays in care will be due to fear, finances, or time constraints. In most cases, the patient's reason for not returning to the previous dentist is dissatisfaction—an inability to have problems resolved—along with perceptions that the previous office could not accommodate his or her schedule, his or her financial demands, or the rejection of an existing or new dental insurance plan. When a patient leaves a practice because of a change of insurance, I can assure you that the previous practice did not develop a strong doctor-patient relationship. Pay attention because the same will happen to you and your practice. I cannot tell you how many times I have heard, "You are the only dentist I will ever see; your practice is the best," followed by, "I am sorry to have to leave your practice now that you do not accept my dental insurance plan. My out-of-pocket expense will be greater so I am going to have to change dentists." What the patient is really saying is that the care and service he or she is receiving are not strong enough or the value he or she perceives is not good enough to keep him or her in your practice.

You should next attempt to quantify a patient's pain level using the pain scale of zero to ten, with ten being the worst pain and zero meaning no pain at all. You should also ascertain how long the patient has been suffering with this pain: a day, a week, a month, or longer. Such information reveals something about your patient's personality and thought processes. You should also ask whether the patient is happy with his or her smile and the color, shape, and position of existing teeth.

I recommend a review of the patient's past medical history as the orientation's next step. We all are aware of how critical it is to stay on schedule, and for many patients, their medical histories can be complex. I suggest focusing on the highlights of your patient's current and past medical history. Please do not get me wrong; all aspects of a medical history are important. However, what part of a patient's past medical history really prevents you from a proper examination and developing a treatment plan, which are the true goals of an initial exam?

I suggest you focus on the following.

- Do you have any allergies?
- Are there medications you cannot take?
- What medications are you currently taking, for what reason, and how long have you been on them?
- Do you have any artificial pins, plates, or joints or any kind of heart murmur?

If the answer to the last question is yes, you may need to premeditate prior to care. You should also ask whether your patient wants, if possible, to resolve his or her chief complaint today, on this initial visit, or on a future visit after the above parameters have been determined.

I recommend you shift gears and provide some internal marketing by informing the patient that the chief complaint can and will be addressed and that the dental office is experienced in providing this particular service and care. It is appropriate at this time to address what makes your practice different from other dental practices. Features that may add to the patient's confidence regarding treatment and care with your office include the following:

- early morning and evening availability;
- twenty-four-hour, on-call service;
- acceptance of specific dental plans;
- a wider range of services, such as implant surgery, TMJ, orthodontics, and oral surgery;
- information about sedation options such as oral sedation, inhalation sedation, and IV sedation; and
- any hospital affiliations, groups, or memberships.

The most important point to make is what makes your practice different; what makes it stand out from other dental practices?

The entire orientation process should be completed in less than fifteen minutes. I recommend that patients be asked to arrive at their initial visit thirty minutes prior to the appointment time so that paperwork and orientation can be completed without taking away from clinical chair time or, better yet, be asked to send such information ahead of time so that it may be completed prior to arrival at the office.

At the end of orientation, you should not be embarrassed to explain to Mr. or Ms. Smith that your office is accepting new patients and would greatly appreciate recommendations to your office to your friends and family. Remember, promoting your practice is your responsibility; however, nothing is better and less expensive than when someone else promotes your organization. We refer to these patients as promoters or raving fans. Do not forget: nothing will help your practice grow more than this group of patients.

It is also critical to determine how patients found out about your practice. Was it from family or friends, television, radio, the Internet, the Yellow Pages, a newspaper, or some other source? The ability to document how patients learn about your practice is critical for effective and successful marketing ventures both present and future. The ability to allocate scarce resource dollars toward marketing is very important. You want to make sure your practice is spending money in the most efficient and effective manner possible. At the end of each business year, you must evaluate such data to determine the best allocation options of resources for the best return on your investment.

As the orientation process ends, a handoff should be provided to the doctor, dental assistant, or hygienist to begin the process of initial records.

5. FINANCIAL GUIDELINES

As the orientation process ends, you will need to address your office's financial policies.

FINANCIAL POLICIES

The office's financial policies should be written down and thoroughly understood by all employees, team members, patients, and, in particular, the front-desk coordinator. That policy should entail payment in full before the procedure is started or a retainer of 50 percent down before procedures are started and the balance paid upon completion of care when patients have approved credit and credit history.

You should be able to provide outside financial options, including Care Credit and Wells Fargo and acceptance of Visa, MasterCard, American Express, or Discover, along with any additional options that may be available. Your organization must understand that all such options, except cash and checks, have a cost to them. Please keep in mind that your practice will pay a fee to such companies for the privilege of using sources of credit, and that cost will be between 2 percent to 21 percent. Therefore, they should be used only as a last resort.

I also suggest a note of caution about accepting cash. Unless you have excellent processes and procedures in place, accepting cash can create many difficult issues for you and your team. Although every day you and your team should balance out the money, cash, and checks coming in, cash is impossible to track and very difficult to account for day to day. Over time, you will be confronted with issues surrounding missing cash: was it stolen, misplaced, or accounted for incorrectly? All these issues can create doubt and tension in your office, and I recommend you avoid it if possible. If Mr. or Ms. Smith states they paid you $100 and you only can account for $50, you will understand my reasoning.

All financial arrangements should be written and signed prior to beginning any dental care and treatment. Failure to have a comprehensive, straightforward financial plan for your office will provide nothing but hardship and problems for you and your team.

During discussion of financial arrangements, the issues of dental insurance and medical insurance must be addressed so that both parties are clear on the process and procedures that must take place when treatment is provided. If you find that the majority of your patients are not accepting your treatment plan, you must inquire to find out why. In many instances, understanding the situation is important because your financial arrangements may be too strict, unfair, or unacceptable. You may also want to consider instituting a dental layaway plan for patients who want care and treatment but for whatever financial reason are unable to receive that care directly and who do not have prior approval via soft credit check. A quick test to see how committed a patient is to undergoing care and treatment can be conducted by setting up an account in which the patient sets aside a certain amount of money every month until ready to undergo treatment. In my thirty-plus years of providing dental care, I have almost never seen a patient complete this arrangement. Still, what is important is that you offer it as an option. What it tells your organization is that Mr. or Ms. Smith wants the care but also wants you and your dental practice to assume all the financial risk. I strongly recommend you do not take such a risk. Patients in almost all instances will be unable to complete their financial arrangements with your practice. They will not keep their hygiene recare or recall appointments, and your company will eventually need to write off the balance or take steps toward collection.

This is a nice segue into reviewing your processes and procedures for uncollected balances, which, I assure you, all practices and businesses have to deal with. For unpaid balances of over thirty days, I suggest a polite reminder; after sixty days, a more firm reminder; and after ninety days, an action letter informing the patient in writing that if the unpaid balance is not paid in full or arrangements have not been made to pay off the balance, collection procedures will go into effect. Please be sure before such statements go out that the patient's care and treatment were completed to the proper standard of care, appropriate informed consents were signed, and records or charts were filled out correctly and completely. Also, confirm that financial policies have been signed by the patient and the appropriate doctor or financial coordinator and phone calls in which you or your staff attempted to contact the patient to work out any issues have been documented. Failure to follow these steps will only create problems. In addition, I suggest you consider using certified mail when contacting patients so that they cannot use an excuse such as, "I did not know I owed you any money…I thought I had paid, and the balance was owed by my insurance company!" There will always be an excuse, trust me. However, your team must develop a process and procedure that makes everyone comfortable.

For unpaid balances of less than $100, my office attempts to reactivate the patient and have him or her pay the unpaid balance before additional care and treatment is started (for patients not returning or who cannot be reactivated, we write those balances off).

For patients who have unpaid balances greater than $100, we inform the credit agency about the patient's unpaid balance. This creates a bad or worse credit history for Mr. or Ms. Smith and, at some point when he or she applies for a car loan, rents an apartment, purchases a home, or applies for any loan, a black mark will show up on his or her credit report. Please make sure that when the balance *is* paid off, your organization has a system in place to remove the black mark from the patient's credit report.

Alternatively, sending patients' bills to a collection agency has not been a successful venture in my experience; however, it may be something you want to consider. Remember, if not all procedures (along with checks and balances) are in order, I do not recommend going down such a path.

6. DENTAL RECORDS

A DENTAL RECORD SHOULD consist of a Panorex survey, four to seven vertical and/or horizontal bitewings, and, when indicated, a full-mouth series. When a patient has a history of periodontal disease, a full series of radiographs will be necessary as well as intra- and extraoral photographs. Such photographs should provide: a full face view; a profile view on both right and left sides; a smile view; a view of the upper six to eight front teeth; views of the right and left cuspid; and upper and lower occlusal views.

The record should also contain the worst intraoral condition for the patient (this particular photo should be put into the treatment plan letter for educational and motivational reasons); upper and lower impressions with centric occlusion bite and, if indicated, a centric relation bite; complete and comprehensive periodontal charting; and an overall assessment of the patient's chief complaint and dental IQ.

I know that there is a debate on whether complete and comprehensive records should be collected on every patient. Let me be clear that there should be virtually no exceptions to this rule. If we look at the problems and complaints expressed by our patient base, in most cases we find that emergency care and service was performed prior to taking comprehensive records. This situation creates both potential and real problems for you and your organization down the road. If the patient does elect to register a complaint against the doctor and/or the dental office, there is no better protection than comprehensive records; they should always be done, regardless of the patient's issue.

7. Treatment Plan

After recording and evaluating comprehensive dental records, a treatment plan must be formulated. Keep in mind that the patient's chief complaint and reason for seeking care and service must be addressed first in most cases. I am well aware that from a clinical standpoint, we sometimes have to bend this directive, but it is imperative that you understand the patient's chief complaint and state that you will be addressing it immediately or in the near future.

I recommend that all treatment plans start with an evaluation of the patient's TMJ. I suggest documenting range of motion. Normal will be forty-five to fifty-five millimeters vertically with no deviations or deflections upon opening or closing; lateral movement to the right and left in a range of four to six millimeters; and protrusive movement four to six millimeters. I also recommend documenting any popping, clicking, or crepitus upon movement and if such sounds occur early or late in the vertical movement evaluation. I also suggest testing the TMJ for loading and checking whether the patient has any pain or tension in either TMJ joint upon loading. You should also ask about any pain in the TMJ area, along with any significant headaches or pattern of headaches. I suggest you evaluate any wear patterns on the teeth and/or a history of grinding or bruxism. A yes in response to any of these exams should sound an alarm for doctors before starting any dental care. Trust me on this. If the TMJ is not healthy, all dental care will suffer, and your life will be much more difficult.

Soft-tissue evaluation will come next. I recommend patients be on a three-, four-, six-, or twelve-month recall for routine hygiene appointments and recare. For patients with significant soft-tissue disease—either gingivitis or periodontitis—I recommend considering a combination of mechanical and chemical intervention that will include root planning, scaling, and prescriptions such as PerioGuard, PreviDent, and Periostat. For individuals allergic to penicillin products, I suggest 250 mg of tetracycline four times a day for thirty days instead of Periostat. For those who smoke more than a half a pack of cigarettes a day, I suggest substituting TheraSol for PerioGuard to avoid staining on the teeth.

Please review the following since, in my opinion, most general dental offices fail to identify and treat lack of attached tissue, furcation involvement, and periodontal pockets greater than five millimeters that bleed upon probing. I then recommend focusing on teeth with a poor long-term prognosis, in particular wisdom teeth. If in doubt, I strongly recommend a treatment plan for removal; whether the patient agrees on such extractions is not as important as the fact that he or she has a treatment plan for removal. This provides documentation that the patient was informed. The patient can never state that he or she did not know that having the wisdom teeth removed when he or she was younger would have less postoperative side effects. We know that as individuals approach age forty-five and beyond, particularly for white females but really for any individual, he or she may require bisphosphonates or antiosteoporotic medication. Remember, surgical intervention in the oral cavity is a potential contraindication due to osteonecrosis. Protect yourself and your practice by having documentation showing these issues have been discussed and reviewed with the patient.

As you focus on other teeth, I suggest that short of a successful prognosis, if the care and treatment of a particular tooth will be less than three to five years, the dentist should consider removing those teeth. This way, Mr. or Ms. Smith cannot make the case that if he or she had known the tooth would have to be removed eventually, he or she would not have made an investment in attempting to save it.

The next step is to replace defective restorations and follow up with missing-tooth replacement. Then, formulate a maintenance plan to make sure your patient has proper follow-up treatment.

The next issue concerns how the treatment plan will be provided and over what time frame. Will the treatment be completed in days, weeks, months, or years? You should then address any necessary sedation options. Of course, we all know most patients do not enjoy having invasive dental treatment. In many cases, review of oral, inhalation, and IV sedation or general anesthesia maybe necessary for a fair number of your patients.

In order to provide an excellent treatment plan, you must have an excellent team. So far, I have covered extensively the front-desk coordinator; now it is time to review the hygiene staff. In my opinion, hygienists are some of a dental office's most highly compensated team members. Yet if you are not careful with your processes and procedures, they may be the most underutilized part of your team for many reasons. Here are some guidelines.

All hygienists should be able to

- take diagnostic photos, impressions, and all types of radiographs (such as Panorex, full-mouth series, vertical and horizontal bitewings, and cephalometric and TMJ radiographs);
- recement temporaries;
- place IRM; and
- discuss and review all risks, benefits, and any alternatives to care and treatment.

They should also be able to

- provide information about fees,
- schedule appointments,

- provide fluoride and local anesthesia,
- place sealants,
- review home-care instructions
- remove sutures,
- place medicaments such as Atridox and Arestin
- perhaps most important, communicate with, educate, and inform patients before you preform in order to improve their dental health.

Too often, hygiene teams lock into a thirty-, forty-, fifty-, or sixty-minute schedule, whether patients need that time or not. Often, they are only providing scaling, not educating patients about differences in care when it comes to scaling versus root planning. Hygienists' lack of multitasking skills negatively affects efficiency in scheduling and production. To improve the situation, make sure your team is on board with expectations and that they buy into your vision. When you are sure your hygiene team is on board, I strongly recommend the appointment of a dedicated assistant to help review and update patients' medical history, update radiographs, provide fluoride treatment and prophy, and seat, drape, and prepare patients for treatment and discharge.

In addition, you must be able to allow your hygiene team an additional operatory. The team must be able to work together and respect one another's skills. Failure to establish teamwork at the outset will only create problems. Teamwork allows your organization to schedule much more effectively, including side scheduling.

Speaking of scheduling issues, horizontal scheduling trumps vertical scheduling. When it comes to children under the age of ten, families who want multiple appointments scheduled on the same day, individuals without a full complement of teeth, and individuals with a history of broken or last-minute cancelations, offices should consider side scheduling. Let us start with children. Anyone who has young children knows they cannot stay seated in a dental chair for forty to sixty minutes. It makes no sense, and, in fact, anything more than twenty minutes is quite inefficient. For those individuals seeking to schedule the whole family, such as a mom and two or three children, we know that if one of them has to cancel, they all cancel, wasting an enormous amount of production time. For individuals with less than a full complement of teeth, is it necessary to schedule forty to sixty minutes to clean two to six teeth? I do not think so.

My opinion is that if patient hygiene is so bad that more than thirty minutes of teeth scaling is needed, then the patient should be on a more frequent hygiene recall recare program, which is a patient issue, not an office issue. In other words, if patients do not wish to be seen more frequently, that is their issue, not ours. It seems to me that in the case of a patient unwilling to be seen more often, in most cases because of cost, the dental office should not have to take a financial hit if the patient will not or cannot take care of hygiene issues.

In each of these cases, scheduling side by side rather than vertically and staggering side books by ten-minute intervals will increase your production and efficiency greatly. I suggest considering such processes and procedures, and that whatever you are paying your hygienist, you might consider that he or she is often able to collect at least three to five times that amount on a daily basis. Therefore, if your hygienist is making $200 per day, he or she should be collecting $600–$1,000 per day. As a general rule, considering my many years of practicing dental medicine and owning a dental office, I suggest that a balanced general dental office is crucial and that the hygiene department should make up about 25 percent to 30 percent of total revenue.

Your hygienist, in most instances, is very concerned with patient oral health and developing a high level of care and service. The issue becomes effectively communicating to your hygiene team the business aspects of being a dental hygienist. I guess if I had my wish, I would want every dental hygienist to be an independent contractor or be an independent hygienist for some time because I feel that would convince them immediately to implement most if not all of these processes and procedures.

The next set of team members charged with making sure your treatment plans are implemented is the dental assistants. In my opinion, these individuals give your dental office the biggest bang for the buck. In most cases, they are the hardest workers, receiving the least yet deserving the highest compensation. A well-trained dental assistant will generate the most revenue of all for your practice's team members provided you are willing to implement the correct processes and procedures. Such professionals are integral to your practice. They should be able to

- set up and break down the dental operatory,
- review treatment plans,
- take all radiographs,
- perform all charting and dental records,
- provide home-care instructions and patient education,
- make and insert temporaries,
- place sealants,
- prophy teeth,
- provide fluoride,
- monitor and take blood pressure and pulse,
- review past medical history, and
- update new medical history.

Dental assistants should have an extensive knowledge of sterilization and infection control as well as a strong working relationship with the doctor, wherein they like, believe, and trust in him or her. They must be dedicated, hardworking, thick-skinned, and great team players. Mutual respect between dental assistants and doctors is essential. Please do not discount this relationship. Your patients will notice and feel such mutual respect and be able to know when the team is working well together.

The next team member to consider might be called a manager, team leader, office facilitator, or point person. In truth, I do not care what you call these individuals. My personal experience is that whenever you give a position a title, in most cases it causes more problems and issues. In any case, you must understand that there is a big difference between management and leadership. In the best of circumstances, if you find an individual who possesses both qualities—he or she is a good manager *and* a leader—you will have hit a homerun. In my opinion, the biggest difference is that managers focus on numbers and orders, and they review the daily, monthly, and yearly reports. They focus on getting better production and collections, and they implement processes and procedures as appropriate. Leaders, meanwhile, set the goals and vision for your organization; they provide the blueprint for your managers to follow. Please do not mix up the two groups. In order to have an excellent team that provides high-quality care and service, you must have both excellent leadership and management.

In small dental practices, you may be looking for someone who possesses both skills. We often assume that would be the owner of the dental practice. In most instances, though, owners will be the least likely individual, having the least amount of time and, in many cases, the least amount of leadership and management experience. Nonetheless, leaders will become obvious to most businesspeople: they rise above, and they put their people and patients ahead of themselves. Your team and patients will gravitate to them in times of crisis. They take responsibility when things don't work out, and they provide credit to others, rather than themselves, when things do work out. When you find a leader, do whatever you can to hold on to him or her. They are rare.

I suggest you consider these reports:

- Net production;
- Net collection;
- How many new patients enter into the practice each month and where they come from;
- How many patients are lost each month and the reason for their leaving;
- Accounts receivable;
- A list of all patients who have not made a payment in more than ninety days;
- A list of all patients who have not kept hygiene recare appointments so they can be followed up and rescheduled; and
- A list of all broken and last-minute cancelations.

Production and collection reports for each provider are important to make sure you are tracking progress and making sure numbers are improving, not just staying the same or decreasing, which is evidence of problems.

8. TMJ

Let's start with background information. TMJ stands for temporal mandibular joint. It is a catchall phrase used particularly by the lay public, expressing to physicians and dentists the presence of pain in or around the ears, head, and neck region or in opening and closing the mouth. Patients may also have a limited range of motion or popping/clicking upon the mouth opening or closing. Many patients will want to be treated by a TMJ specialist. You must first make clear that in the strict meaning of the term and in the fields of dentistry and medicine, there is no such thing. One cannot graduate from medical or dental school with a specialty degree in TMJ. There are, however, individuals with great interests in the subject who have received additional training related to enhancing their knowledge and skills in providing care and treatment for patients who suffer from TMJ and its signs and symptoms.

First, you must follow the processes and procedures as follows. Take a history and examination from your patient. I provide documentation for this at the end of this book. Next, document your patient's ROM (range of motion) vertically, laterally, and protrusive. During this evaluation, document whether your patient has any deviations or deflections. A deviation occurs when your patient opens vertically, and his or her lower jaw moves to the right or left and does not return to the midline. A deflection is when the lower jaw moves to the right or left upon opening but then drifts toward the midline. The next step is palpation of the muscles of mastication to determine if such muscles are tender or not. Next, you should acquire the radiographic workup along with diagnostic impressions and bite. You should finish this procedure with a written report of your findings and diagnosis.

Now let's look at each of these procedures in more depth. Your patient's symptoms will include the following:

- Cephalgia, or pain around the head area
- Photophobia, or painful symptoms related to light, dizziness, or light-headedness
- Tinnitus, or ringing in the ears
- Sinus issues, such as postnasal drip
- Popping or clicking upon opening of the mouth
- Crepitus, a grating sound in the TMJ upon opening or closing
- Difficulty opening and closing the mouth
- Difficulty chewing or swallowing
- Chronic sore throat, stiff neck, and shoulder pain

I recommend asking patients about these issues, including questions related to how long they've had such signs and symptoms, and documenting whether they feel they need treatment. For example, "On a pain scale from zero to ten, with ten being the worst pain possible, how would you quantify your pain level?" Any of these signs or symptoms could indicate that your patient is suffering from TMJ issues.

Next, document range of motion. Vertically, measure from incisal papilla on the maxilla to papilla on the mandible; normal should be forty to fifty-five millimeters with no deviations or deflections. Laterally, measure from the maxillary midline to the mandibular central incisal papilla as the patient moves his or her jaw all the way left and right. Normal will be between six to ten millimeters. Protrusive range of motion is next, in which you ask the patient to move his or her lower jaw as far as possible forward and measure from maxillary papilla to mandibular papilla. Using the papilla instead of the teeth allows you to take measurements even when the patient is edentulous. Keep in mind when you are examining ROM that you should also document any popping, clicking, or crepitus, as well as whether such noises take place early, middle, or late during openings or closings.

Next is palpation of the major muscles of mastication, such as the temporalis muscle and its three portions (anterior, middle, and posterior); the masseter muscle; the sternocleidomastoid muscle; and the medial and lateral pterygoid muscles.

Keep in mind that muscles associated with opening the mouth are digastric, mylohyoid, geniohyoid, and the inferior head of the lateral pterygoid. Muscles associated with closing the mouth are the temporalis, masseter, medial pterygoid, and the superior head of the lateral pterygoid. Lateral excursions are caused by the posterior portion of the ipsilateral temporalis, the contralateral medial pterygoid, and the inferior head of the contralateral external pterygoid. Protrusion is caused by the masseters, medial pterygoids, suprahyoids, and the inferior head of the lateral pterygoids. Retrusion is caused by the posterior portion of the middle temporalis and the anterior and posterior digastricus.

Some definitions relating to muscle activity are in order. Isometric contraction means an increased tension within a muscle that maintains a constant muscle length. Isotonic contraction produces a shortening in the length of a muscle. Muscle tonus occurs when a muscle has resistance to stretching. Muscle splinting is a temporary state of hypertonicity induced as a protective mechanism to stabilize a threatened body part. It is a normal physiologic protective mechanism and is painful, but the muscle still functions to the normal limits of its range of motion. A muscle spasm is neurologically induced and is involuntary muscle contraction. It is also painful, as the muscle shortens and becomes rigid. Contracture of a muscle associated with internal derangements is shortening of a muscle not allowed to stretch to its full length where there is no neurological input.

What does the click mean? In reality, the meniscus or disc creates the noise. The disc is what is between the condylar head and eminence of the glenoid fossa. It prevents bone from rubbing against bone. Remember that this disc is attached to the condylar head by attaching to the medial and lateral poles of the condyle. As the condyle moves down and forward in normal movement, the disc rotates backward when everything is working well. When this complex is not functioning as described, we refer to the problem as internal derangement of the TMJ. Remember, internal derangement can be temporary, semipermanent, or permanent.

A TMJ that has internal derangement can be classified as reciprocal clicking, meaning dislocation with reduction, further defined as early opening unilateral, midopening unilateral, late opening unilateral, or early, mid, or late opening bilateral.

Intermittent locking is dislocation with reduction, which can be either unilateral or bilateral. Closed locking is dislocation without reduction, which can be broken down to unilateral acute or chronic or bilateral acute or chronic.

When you hear the click, it is the disc actually popping into the correct position. An early click is defined as a click occurring within the first five millimeters of opening or less. A midclick occurs at about twenty-five millimeters, and a late opening click is at about forty-five millimeters of opening.

The later the click, the longer the eminence and condylar head and disc complex are out of position, potentially causing more damage. When you hear no click at all, it simply means the disc never returns to its correct position.

During intermittent locking, you either hear clicking or you don't, and sometimes patients will complain about the jaw being locked. What is really happening, though, is that sometimes the joint is fine and other times it is not. The disc will reduce, sometimes popping into the correct position, but at other times, it is unable to pop into the correct position or it will not reduce. The more frequently this occurs, the worse off your patient will become. In most cases, the patient will regress to an even worse condition known as a closed locked joint.

In the closed locked condition, dislocation occurs without reduction so the disc is always out of place, and it is never interposed between the condyle and eminence. This is the most severe internal derangement condition. What is actually happening in such cases is that the condyle is functioning against the retrodiscal ligament, which is not meant to be load bearing. If this condition has lasted less than six months, we call it acute; if it has lasted more than six months, we call it chronic. When acute, the condition is very painful, and you will see a significant deflection away from the midline on opening. When chronic, the deflection will be less severe from the midline. Under chronic conditions, it is likely that tissue will perforate, allowing bone to rub against bone. The resulting grating sound is called crepitus, and it will cause osseous breakdown or osteoarthritic degeneration. Remember that untreated, clicking will progress to crepitus if the patient lives long enough; it is just a matter of time.

The most common problem seen with internal derangement is bilateral reciprocal clicking, followed by unilateral clicking; in most cases, these will occur on the left side. The third scenario is called intermittent locking joint and is very difficult to diagnosis since sometimes the joint looks and sounds fine. However, you must ask your patient whether the jaw ever locks or becomes stuck.

When the disc is out of position, patients will say they feel their teeth are hitting first on the side in which the disc is out of position. Restoring teeth under these conditions, whether involving restorations with fillings or crowns or even orthodontics, is not a good idea and can lead to severe problems that patients and dentists may not even be aware of. As the condition goes from acute to chronic, you will see on the affected side a depression of teeth, which is noticeable as a more severe Curve of Spee and greater freeway space on the affected side. Simply ask the patient to open his or her mouth and observe the plane of occlusion. Other noticeable signs include fractured restorations, perforation of gold occlusal surfaces, and depression of mandibular posterior teeth, as well as excessive attrition.

What are the treatment goals for patients with TMJ issues?

- A vertical range of motion of at least forty-eight millimeters
- Lateral excursions of twelve millimeters or greater
- No joint noises, deflections, or deviation upon opening
- The condyle translating past the eminence radiographically
- The condyle being separated from the eminence by at least two millimeters on maximum opening radiographically
- No pain in the TMJ area

INFORMATION ABOUT TREATMENT AND CARE FOR YOUR PATIENTS

Appliances or splints—what do they do and why do they work? They can decompress the tissues of the TMJ. They can restore the foreshortened muscles of masticatory muscles to their resting length. They can decrease proprioception to the nervous system. They can limit TMJ functional movements to promote healing. They can decrease electrical activity of muscles. You should understand that other treatment might be necessary for care and treatment, such as ultrasound, TENS, and trigger-point injections, but in most cases, splints will be used to reposition the mandible to a new relationship with the maxilla.

Splint options are as follows:

- For the maxilla, you have smooth surface, central occlusion, pull-forward, distalization of the mandible, and pivot types of splints, as well as palatal expansion and sagittal types.
- For the mandible, you have flat, pull-forward, and pivot.

You must remember that after splint delivery, you must follow up with the patient every three to six weeks for splint adjustments as the TMJ starts to heal and change.

Consider the following guidelines. If the problem is clearly muscular in nature or myalgia and the TMJ is normal with no noises, consider a flat-plane on either the upper or lower arch but the lower first since it will not impede the midpalatal suture. If the patient doesn't respond, then consider an upper splint. In cases where the patient has a unilateral or bilateral reciprocal click that disappears when the mandible is closed anteriorly to the click, consider a pull-forward splint, which should be constructed just anterior to where the click starts. In cases where the patient has a unilateral closed locked type of condition, you first must manipulate the lower jaw, either manually or with a molt retractor with local anesthetic, to get the disc into position; if successful, place a pull-forward splint in. If you cannot accomplish this, you should consider attempting to decompress the tissues of the joint by moving the condyle inferiorly, creating more superior joint space, which will allow the disc to move into position. In conditions where the patient has a bilateral closed locked condition, consider a pivot splint to move the condyles inferiorly. When you start to hear the click, convert the splint to a pull-forward type of splint. Try not to use a flat-plane splint when a patient has a unilateral or bilateral reciprocal clicking joint since this can lead to the joint becoming closed locked.

When constructing the flat-plane splint, it should be on the lower arch, flat, smooth, and about one and a half to two millimeters thick. It should have four dots on either side from occlusal marking made from the lingual cusp of the first and second molars and premolars.

For the pivot type of splint, you want a single point of contact on either side where the mesiopalatal cusp of the maxillary first molars occlude against the flat surface on the mandibular splint in the left and right first-molar areas. The most important part of this splint is not horizontal but vertical dimension. You must keep in mind that this splint must be adjusted every four to six weeks to keep pace with the changes in the TMJ. Remember, this will not be the final vertical dimension but just the start until the issues with the bilateral closed locked joint have been corrected.

You may want to consider three methods to establish your vertical dimension for this pivot type of splint. One is the physiological or swallow approach, where the patient swallows into a mound of soft, red wax prepositioned on the mandibular splint in the first-molar area. You should be aware that other options exist but consider this one.

The pull-forward splint, which is used in reciprocal clicking or unilateral closed lock, is created at a treatment position that allows the patient to open and close the mouth without the disc becoming displaced. This position is usually edge-to-edge but anterior to where the click occurs.

Remember, stage one is getting the patient comfortable and allowing the TMJ to heal. That means the splint will need to be periodically adjusted. Stage two occurs when the patient has the following signs of success: no pain, no noises, no deflections or deviations, a range of motion within normal limits, and normal radiographic images. Keep in mind that after splint therapy, in most cases you will have open-posterior occlusion. When the patient has been symptom-free for six to twelve months, you will then consider stage two, which includes occlusal buildup such as crown and bridge or overdenture prosthetics, orthognathic surgery, or orthodontics. It is critical that your patient understands these phases before you ever start treatment.

I strongly suggest reviewing the work of Dr. Brendan C. Stack, BS, DDS, MS, who has written and published extensively about TMJ and from which the majority of my information and recommendations emanate. In particular, his book *Advanced TMJ Level 1 Diagnosis to Splint Construction* is recommended.

On some occasions, you will find it necessary to do occlusal adjustment. The following are some guidelines to consider. After relieving a patient's symptoms with splint therapy, you may need to consider bite adjustment. First, we must agree that the condyles can rotate to open or close the jaw without moving out of the fully seated position in their respective fossa. Remember, the mandible can be in centric relation even when the teeth are separated. Centric relation should be the starting point. The condyles must not be restricted to centric relation but free to move in and out of centric relation during function. We define centric relation as the relationship of the mandible to the maxilla when the properly aligned condyle disk assemblies are in the most superior position against eminentia, irrespective of vertical dimension or tooth position. When properly aligned, the condyle and disk assembly in centric relation can resist maximum loading by the elevator muscles with no sign of discomfort. Centric relation should not be confused with centric occlusion, which refers to the jaw position during maximum intercuspation of the teeth, regardless of whether the condyles are physiologically seated.

Some considerations for a stable occlusion are the following:

- Stable stops on all teeth of equal intensity when the condyles are in centric relation
- Anterior guidance in harmony with the border movements of the envelope of function
- Disclusion of all posterior teeth in protrusive movements
- Disclusion of all posterior teeth on the nonworking, balancing side
- Disclusion or noninterference of all posterior teeth on the working side with either the lateral anterior guidance or the border movements of the condyle

Anterior guidance (or should I say, proper anterior guidance) is the key. You must first consider mounted models on an appropriate articulator that simulates the patient's arc of closure. When accurate mounting is verified, mark the first contact. Then check lower anterior, occlusal plan, centric relation stops, and anterior guidance. Next, mark hopeless or questionable teeth. Next is to unlock the articulator and go from centric relation to centric occlusion or maximum intercuspation. The distance or space between this and centric relation and first contact is the amount of room available to establish vertical dimension. We then equilibrate all premature interfering contacts. The goal is to have uniform stops all the way around the arch, including anterior teeth, with good cusp fossa relationships on each posterior tooth and a stable holding contact on each anterior tooth. If that is not possible, move teeth or wax up on teeth to achieve this goal, starting with lower anterior teeth. You next eliminate all balancing and working interferences. Then recheck anterior guidance again to make sure you have an acceptable envelope of function. When this is completed, you should be able to visualize whether the treatment can be completed through equilibration or if you need to reposition or restore teeth to create occlusal stability.

If, after evaluation of models, it is deemed that equilibration can be done, consider the following. First, load test to make sure the TMJ area is comfortable. Then begin to adjust to centric relation stops with high speed and develop cusp-to-fossa contacts on posterior teeth. When adjusting on the lower teeth, consider using slow speed. When all stops in centric relation look good and the patient states he or she does not feel any teeth touching before another tooth as they are tapped together, then make sure the patient's front teeth do not touch before his or her back teeth. Consider using black articulator paper on centric relation stops and red articulator marks for excursive movements. Lastly, polish all teeth so they are smooth. Remember to recheck the patient at follow-up appointments to make sure the patient is comfortable, all contacts are equal, and there is no pain to the TMJ upon loading.

In many cases, the average patient will need two or three additional follow-up appointments to make sure occlusion is stable. We can measure success by the following:

- When load testing, the TMJ is comfortable.
- The patient can clench teeth together without pain.
- The patient has comfort on all occlusal function.

I would like to thank Dr. Peter Dawson and suggest the reader review his book *Evaluation, Diagnosis, and Treatment of Occlusal Problems*, second edition. I would also like to like to thank Dr. Glenn E. DuPont and his study guide, *A Predictable Step-By-Step Approach to Occlusal Equilibration*.

9. PERIODONTICS

Let's keep it simple: almost all patients have some type of periodontal disease. Gingivitis, where inflammation is confined to the soft tissue, involves no bone loss. Periodontitis, on the other hand, means bone loss. Whenever you have periodontitis, you also have gingivitis, but just because you have gingivitis does not mean you have periodontitis. The diseases can be classified as follows:

- Type one: gingivitis-inflamed tissue, no bone loss
- Type two: early periodontitis with mild bone loss but without furcation involvement
- Type three: moderate periodontitis with moderate bone loss and early furcation involvement
- Type four: periodontitis or advanced periodontitis, which involves severe bone loss and extensive furcation invasion

Bacteria, which are mostly Gram-negative, combined with cell walls that have a lipopolysaccharide base or endotoxin that causes inflammation cause the disease. The bacteria are anaerobic and can be motile or nonmotile. The generally accepted bacteria that cause periodontal disease are *Actinobacillus actinomycetemcomitans*, *Fusobacterium nucleatum*, *Peptostreptococcus micros*, *Porphyromonas gingivalis*, *Prevotella intermedia/nigresens*, *Tannerella forsythia*, and *Treponema denticola*.

Some risk factors associated with periodontal issues are exposed furcation, bifurcated ridges, cervical enamel projections, palatogingival grooves, open contacts, accessory root canals, overhanging restorations, and violation of the biological width, which means the dental restoration is less than three millimeters from the bone level, causing inflammation. Others include occlusal traumatism, diabetes mellitus, HIV/AIDS, smoking, sex hormone imbalance, and genetic predisposition. In 1999, the American Academy of Periodontology (AAP) elected to provide a more descriptive system for periodontal disease.

What should you look for? First, when was the patient's last visit and why? What this tells you is the patient's dental IQ. Unless the patient has avoided the dental office for a particularly good reason, dealing with a patient who does not go to the dentist will be an uphill battle when treating periodontal disease. If you see in the patient history that your subject smokes a half pack of cigarettes a day or more along with consuming alcohol every day, you will have an uphill battle. You should also look at your patient's hygiene: is it good, fair, or bad? If it's bad, you will have an uphill battle. This really becomes a risk assessment. The higher the risk, the poorer the outcome you can expect.

To quantify such a risk, look at the number of missing teeth, decayed teeth, and teeth with restorations. Any patient with more than ten—excluding wisdom teeth and missing premolars due to orthodontic care—should signal a red flag. You will have an uphill battle resolving your patient's periodontal disease. Check plaque score—i.e., how many surfaces of the teeth with plaque compared to no plaque. Next, look at bleeding score or for bleeding upon probing, which is likely the best indicator of inflammation. Next, look at periodontal pocketing greater than five millimeters with bleeding.

You should then evaluate recession and the attached gingiva. For recession, it is just the distance from the free-gingival margin to the CEJ (cemental enamel junction). Attached gingiva is simply the amount of keratinized tissue on the buccal and facial of the upper arch and buccal, facial, and lingual surfaces of the lower arch. Both recession and lack of attached gingiva is important if you have a patient who is sensitive to temperature, planning orthodontic care, planning on restorations on the teeth with recession and lack of attached gingiva, or bothered by the appearance of his or her teeth from an esthetic standpoint.

You must also consider furcation involvement where you have a grade one, two, three, or four lesion. Grade one is simply incipient bone loss in the furcation area. Grade two is partial bone loss. Grade three is total bone loss with a through-and-through opening of the furcation that is not visible. Grade four is through-and-through bone loss that is visible.

Lastly, consider mobility from zero to three, with zero meaning no mobility, one meaning mobility is perceptible, two meaning mobility that is less than one millimeter faciolingually but containing no apical movement, and three meaning apical movement as well as lateral movement. A note of caution: when the above reading is present, the prognosis of the tooth and/or dentition is questionable, and you will have a guarded prognosis. I have found that in many patients, if they do not have pain and cannot visualize the disease process, motivation to seek care and treatment and achieve long-term success is minimal. Please don't get me wrong. I suggest you create a treatment plan, diagnose the problem, and recommend care, but in the long term it will be an uphill battle. In fact, most patients will blame the provider and never consider the problem to be theirs. I shouldn't say this but I sometimes do: "Mr. or Ms. Smith, if God gave you thirty-two teeth and you have lost some, trust me, no matter what treatment we consider, you will be fighting an uphill battle."

I have always looked at periodontal disease as similar to weight problems. The majority of patients with weight issues will diet, but very few stick to the diet and even fewer keep the weight off in the long term. In my experience, what I often see in periodontal disease is short-term success and long-term failure. Please be aware when electing to care for and treat periodontal conditions that you must communicate clearly with your patients, making sure they understand that the majority of the success depends on his or her ability to keep appointments and follow excellent home-care and hygiene programs. Also, remember that with so many third-party payers, your patient will need a series of full-mouth radiographs so that you and your patient's insurance carrier can see bone loss interproximally.

Depending on your patient's risk factors, I suggest considering the following options for care: mechanical treatment, chemical treatment, surgical treatment, or some combination of the three. Mechanical treatment is root planning, scaling, and a recall entailing one, two, or three months for periodontal maintenance. Please keep in mind that if your patient needs mechanical care, you should factor in chemical treatment also. Chemical treatment involves medicaments such as Periostat, PerioGuard, and PreviDent, or what I refer to as the three P's. I also suggest you consider the use of Arestin in this group. Consider the following medications for three to six months and then reevaluate:

- Metronidazole, 500 milligrams TID (three times daily) for eight days
- Clindamycin, 300 milligrams TID for eight days
- Doxycycline or minocycline, 100–200 milligrams QD (once daily) for twenty-one days
- Ciprofloxacin, 500 milligrams BID (twice daily) for eight days
- Azithromycin, 500 mg QD for four to seven days
- Metronidazole plus amoxicillin, 250 milligrams TID for eight days of each drug
- Metronidazole plus ciprofloxacin, 500 milligrams BID for eight days of each drug

The exception, though, is the following: if your patient is allergic to penicillin products, consider tetracycline 250 milligrams Q6H (every six hours) for twenty-eight days. If your patient is a heavy smoker, consider substituting TheraSol for PerioGuard to reduce heavy staining.

After this phase of care, reevaluate the patient and consider whether periodontal surgery would be beneficial or ineffective. Every day a patient tells me he or she has had periodontal surgery, and it has not worked. In my opinion, the treatment is done properly but often on the wrong type of patient—with high risks and poor long-term prognosis. That does not mean you should not attempt periodontal surgery, but you should communicate very clearly that the long-term prognosis is often poor and that additional care will be necessary. Write this down and do not forget it.

The third option for periodontal care and treatment is surgery. Its goal is to reduce or eliminate periodontal pocketing that has not responded to mechanical and chemical care and to correct or reduce tissue recession and/or the lack of attached gingiva. The last option for the surgical phase would be cosmetic. So many times, we consider restorative treatment without considering the height of the free-gingival margin. What happens in cases like these is that after the veneers and/or crowns have been placed, the height or length of teeth looks different to your patient due to failing to address the free-gingival margin height before treatment starts. Please address this first, not after care has been completed. Lastly regarding periodontal surgery, consider before you place any restoration where the margin of the restoration will be in proximity to the bone level on the tooth. As a rule of thumb, keep your restorative margin three to five millimeters from the bone level. When this fails to happen, communicate with your patient about the need for crown lengthening; ideally, do this before you perform the restoration, not after.

I recommend if considering periodontal surgery, you divide the mouth into six sections—upper right, upper front, upper left, lower right, lower front, and lower left—or into sextants. For the beginner, I recommend avoiding the upper-front sextant six to eleven until you have gained experience. The decision to consider in the surgical phase is your incision, keeping the following in mind: if your patient lacks attached gingiva, consider an intrasulcular incision; if your patient has adequate attached gingiva, consider an extrasulcular incision. Next, decide whether you are planning to address any bony defects or need to reposition the tissue. Let's assume you're not, so no vertical releasing incisions will be needed.

Simply retract your flap and root plane and scale and suture up. If you do need to address the bone or reposition your flap, remember you will need vertical releasing incisions and the base of your flap should be wider at the apical portion for blood supply. In such cases, you will again root plane and scale and then address the bony issues, starting by creating positive architecture, which simply means keeping the interproximal bone higher than the buccal and lingual bone and then deciding whether bone grafting will be beneficial or not and whether the recontouring of the bone will be necessary.

In the end, you must suture the area with a continuous sling suture to reposition tissue. This simply means you suture the buccal and/or facial flap and then the lingual area. The sling suture is done by first pass to the buccal and first puncture is on the lingual so the knot will be on the facial. You're making your puncture on the lingual, going interproximal between each tooth, and making the puncture on the lingual, not the labial, so that the lingual tissue is held by the buccal and facial teeth. As you go to the most distal tooth in the sextant, make punctures on the facial and wrap around the lingual, continuing until you meet the tail of your suture, and tie off on the facial. In no way do I want to diminish the skill and difficulty required of periodontal surgery or of any other care, but in the end the goal is to keep the teeth clean and free from plaque and calculus. Continue to follow up with the patient for routine hygiene visits.

A few comments about bone fill and regeneration of the periodontium and when membranes are called for: it appears they all work; the goal of any barrier is simply to prevent the invagination of soft tissue into the wound, which will disrupt your graft or healing process and allows less pocket reduction than hoped. Keep in mind if you use a membrane, whether is it resorbable or not, you should attempt primary closure if possible to reduce infection and promote healing. Some examples of nonresorbable membranes are PTFE (polytetrafluoroethylene) or resorbable membranes, such as collagen-based membranes, which would be BioMend type one, resolute type one, or polymer-based membranes such as Atrisorb (which is polyactic acid), and others such as CAPSET, which is calcium sulfate or plaster of Paris.

When considering bone-graft materials, you have autograft (grafts taken from one part of an individual and placed into another part of the same individual, such as an extraction site), exostoses, or edentulous ridge. You also have allograft, which is a graft between genetically dissimilar members of the same species, the main types of which are freeze-dried and demineralized freeze-dried. Alloplast graft is a synthetic or inert foreign graft in which some of the materials are resorbable and some are not. Please keep in mind that if you're considering a dental implant in the future, you may not want to place an alloplastic nonresorbable graft in that site. A xenograft is a graft taken from a different species, such as bovine (cow) or porcine (pig).

Always remember risk factors when considering any treatment, but in particular with periodontics and endodontic.

When considering recession of gingiva, Sullivan and Atkins have a classification for recession, comprised of shallow and narrow, deep and narrow, shallow and wide, and deep and wide. Shallow and narrow has the best prognosis. Miller also has a classification system, class I, which states recession is coronal to MGJ and no interproximal bone loss. Class II recession is apical to MGJ with no interproximal bone loss. Class III recession is apical to MGJ and mild interproximal bone loss. Class IV recession is apical to MGJ and severe interproximal bone loss. Within these classifications, I and II should be very successful, whereas classes III and IV will have a poor prognosis for root coverage.

Consider the following problems and possible solutions.

1. **Gingival recession or inadequate zone of attached gingiva**: the solution would be free-gingival graft, submucosal connective tissue graft, lateral pedicle graft, alloderm graft, or a coronally positioned flap.
2. **Inadequate zone of attached gingiva without recession:** your options would be a free-gingival graft or alloderm graft.
3. **To prevent ridge resorption**, consider socket preservation or retention of teeth or roots.
4. **For the resorption of the edentulous ridge**, you may want to consider submucosal connective tissue graft, onlay connective tissue graft, particulate bone graft, guided bone regeneration, or distraction osteogenesis.
5. **For aberrant frenum**, consider frenectomy.
6. **For excessive gingival display**, consider gingivectomy or crown lengthening or orthognathic surgery.

Some additional periodontal issues that you may need to address include:

1. **For periodontal abscess**, consider establishing drainage to relieve pressure, consider tooth removal, depending on the support that is remaining, and consider antibiotics.
2. **For pericoronitis**, consider occlusal adjustment if the opposing tooth is interfering, antibiotics, and removal of partially impacted tooth.

The difference between diagnosis of a periodontal abscess and an endodontic abscess is that pain for an endodontic lesion tends to be sharp and more rapid in onset, but the periodontal abscess is more diffuse or throbbing in nature. The probing depth tends to be wider with periodontal abscess; I suggest you place a size-thirty gutta-percha cone to trace the fistula or pocket. Pulpal vitality will be problematic in making a diagnosis. In most cases, treat the pulp with endodontic problems first and then address the periodontal tissue second. Keep in mind that with a poor prognosis, you will be better off removing the tooth.

10. ENDODONTIC

THE PULP INSIDE the tooth has been damaged. It will get better or not. If it does not, we will extract the tooth or start root-canal care and treatment. The pulp's primary functions are the formation of tubular dentin, nutritional support for avascular dentin, protection of the tooth by giving dentin its sensitivity, and the repair of dentin. The pulp can be damaged by bacteria invasion, trauma, or both, and thought should be given to the long-term prognosis of the tooth. For most patients, spending a lot of money and time only to have the tooth removed usually leads to dissatisfaction. Also, make sure your patients fully understand before care and treatment that in most cases the tooth will need a buildup and crown, requiring additional visits and costs. Again, this discussion should occur before you perform, not after. Please make sure you have a preoperative radiograph showing the apex and clinical crown along with adjacent teeth before you begin the care. I also suggest informing the patient before starting that around 8 percent of all root canals fail no matter what strategy is attempted; that is simply a risk of treatment.

Let's start with primary teeth. In general, I suggest you only focus on cuspids and first and second molars. Please remember to inform parents that the reason for attempting to save primary teeth that will be lost in the future are many; however, perhaps most the most important reason is to save leeway space, allowing for the proper eruption of permanent teeth. If you elect to remove the primary cuspid, consider bilateral extractions to avoid midline shifts. If removing primary first and second molars, consider a fixed-space maintainer to hold space. Remember to review with parents beforehand since many times parents will make a decision for the less-expensive extraction, failing to realize their son or daughter will need additional care, which means additional costs.

Pulp capping, whether direct or indirect, with calcium hydroxide should only be done when one millimeter or less of the pulp is exposed. If greater exposure is present, in most cases calcium hydroxide will cause internal resorption. For the more extensive pulp exposure of primary teeth, consider Formo Cresol, which is a medicament made of 19 percent formaldehyde, 35 percent tricresol, and 15 percent glycerin in water. In contrast to calcium hydroxide, Formo Cresol does not stimulate the healing of remaining vital tissue. Formo Cresol, while very toxic, kills bacteria and fixes tissue.

INDIRECT PULP TREATMENT ON PRIMARY TEETH

This occurs when, in cases involving deep caries, there is danger of exposing the pulp if all the caries are removed. You should remove the bulk of carious tissue and leave a small amount of carious dentin in the deepest area of the cavity. Place a bactericidal medicament such calcium hydroxide over that area and then a temporary restoration.

Several weeks later, usually eight to twelve weeks, retreat the tooth by removing the remainder of the decay and restore with a final restoration. Keep in mind, not everyone in the dental community will agree with this technique for primary teeth. Many practitioners will recommend complete removal of caries and, if the pulp is exposed, proceed to pulpotomy.

Some contraindications of this technique would be radiographic evidence of probable or definite pulp exposure, evidence of calcified masses in the pulpal horn area, thickening of the periodontal membrane, or if the patient is experiencing prolonged spontaneous pain in the tooth. Other conditions include mobility, sensitivity to percussion, and swollen and sore surrounding soft tissue.

DIRECT PULP CAPPING ON PRIMARY TEETH

This is a method of vital pulp therapy used when a rotary or hand instrument causes a pinpoint mechanical exposure of the pulp during cavity preparation. The technique entails simply drying and cleaning the area and then placing calcium hydroxide in the usual manner and place for planned restoration.

Contraindications to this method include radiographic evidence of pulpal degeneration. The patient may experience prolonged spontaneous pain in the tooth, swollen and red surrounding soft tissue, excessive mobility, mechanical exposure greater than one millimeter in diameter, or multiple exposures or excessive hemorrhaging at the exposure site (bleeding fails to stop after three to five minutes); or you may notice pus. Please make sure the patient and the patient's family understand that extraction or a root canal may be needed down the road.

FORMO CRESOL PULPOTOMY FOR PRIMARY TEETH

This method may be the most widely accepted treatment for carious or traumatic pulp exposures in primary teeth. When this situation occurs, in most cases the pulp in the crown portion will be inflamed; however, the pulp in the root portion may be perfectly fine. In such cases, the coronal pulp is removed or amputated, the remaining pulp is fixed with Formo Cresol-soaked cotton pellets for five minutes, and then a layer of zinc oxide eugenol is placed and the tooth is restored, in most cases with a stainless-steel crown.

Contraindication to this method include radiographic evidence of pathologic bone loss or internal resorption, calcified masses in the pulpal horn area, widening of the PDL or periodontal ligament, spontaneous pain, pus, excessive mobility, or swelling around the soft tissue. You should also consider the usefulness of the tooth. Its remaining roots should be at least two-thirds still present, and the tooth should be able to last at least another twelve months before it would be exfoliated on its own.

PULPECTOMY ON PRIMARY TEETH

This is used on primary teeth in which the pulp is nonvital or the infected pulp has spread beyond the coronal pulp tissue. In these cases, the entire pulp is removed from the coronal and radicular areas. You should first amputate the coronal pulp and then instrument the radicular pulp tissue going one-half to one millimeter from the apex. Then irrigate with hydrogen peroxide and follow up with sodium hypochlorite, dry with paper points, fill with zinc oxide eugenol, and restore with a stainless-steel crown.

Contraindications to this procedure include radiographic evidence of extensive periapical destruction, two-thirds of the root's length or less remaining, or pathologic resorption or pus coming from the area.

PERMANENT DENTITION

For this, let us first review common access and canal configurations.

Maxillary central incisors

These are single root, are usually straight, and usually have only one canal, with a length of twenty-three to twenty-five millimeters. They erupt around age seven to eight, and the chamber is triangular in design. Remember during access to remove the lingual edge.

Maxillary lateral incisors

These are single root, usually one canal, and usually twenty-two to twenty-three millimeters in length. The curve is usually toward the distal and palatal, erupting around age seven to nine, and the chamber is similar to the maxillary central incisor except smaller.

Maxillary canine

These are single root, usually one canal, and twenty-four to twenty-seven millimeters in length. They erupt around age eleven, and the chamber is elliptical or oval and will usually have a lingual ledge.

Maxillary first premolar

This will be a single- or two-rooted system; root fusion can occur, usually two canals—buccal and palatal about 85 percent of the time. When there are two roots, the tooth usually has separate foramens, and the palatal root is usually larger and longer (typical length twenty-one to twenty-two millimeters). The tooth usually erupts around age ten to eleven. The chamber shape is oval.

Maxillary second premolar

This is usually a single- or two-rooted system, but in most cases it's single, with one canal, with a length around twenty-one to twenty-two millimeters. It erupts around age ten to twelve, and the chamber is oval.

Maxillary first molar

This is usually a three-rooted system but will frequently have four canals with mesial-buccal root, distal-buccal root, and palatal root, with the mesial-buccal root having a high likelihood of having two canals—a mesial-buccal and mesial-palatal canal. The tooth will erupt around age six to seven, the chamber is triangular to square, and access should be distal to the mesial marginal ridge.

Maxillary second molar

This is usually a three-rooted system, with a mesial-buccal, distal-buccal, and palatal root, with the mesial-buccal root sometimes having two canals. Typical length is nineteen to twenty-two millimeters, the chamber shape is less triangular and more oval, and it will usually erupt around age twelve to thirteen.

Mandibular central and lateral incisors

These have a high probability of two canals, facial and lingual, with a common orifice. Typical length is twenty-one to twenty-two millimeters. These teeth usually erupt around age six to eight. The chamber is triangular to oval and will often have a lingual edge.

Mandibular canine

This is usually a single root with one canal. Typical length is twenty-five to twenty-six millimeters. It erupts around age nine to ten, and the chamber is oval.

Mandibular first premolar

This is usually a single root with one canal with a length of twenty-one to twenty-two millimeters. They erupt around age ten to twelve, and the chamber is oval.

Mandibular second premolar

This is usually a single root, with a length of twenty-one to twenty-two millimeters. It erupts around age eleven to twelve, and it has an oval chamber.

Mandibular first molar

This is usually a two-rooted system, a mesial and distal. In many cases the mesial root will have two canals, but the distal root may also have two canals. Typical length is twenty-one to twenty-three millimeters. It erupts around age six to seven, and the chamber is triangular to square.

Mandibular second molar

This is usually a two-rooted system. It will have a length of twenty to twenty-one millimeters. It erupts around age eleven to thirteen, and the chamber is triangular.

DIAGNOSIS OF DENTAL PULP

Consider the following steps. Find your patient's chief complaint, review your patient's past and current medical history, document your patient's subjective symptoms, try to reproduce your patient's symptoms, and perform any additional tests that can help with diagnosis. Then make your diagnosis and provide appropriate care and treatment.

When reviewing pain, consider the following: what is stimulating the pain? Is it chewing, cold, or heat? What are the frequency, duration, and severity of the pain? Does the pain occur spontaneously or not?

Temperature tests such as cold can be done by using several different components: Endo-Ice (Hygenic Corp.), CO2 ice (Moyco Union Broach), Frigi-Dent (Ellman), ice, or ethyl chloride, although the latter two may be more unreliable than the other options. When testing with heat, consider a Burlew disc on slow speed, a heated compound stick, or an endodontic irrigating syringe filled with hot water. With both cold and heat testing, consider isolating the tooth with a rubber dam and waiting for one to two minutes between testing each tooth for the best results.

A normal pulp will have little or no sensitivity to heat or cold; if the tooth does have a response, that response will last only three to ten seconds. A pulp with reversible pulpitis will usually have a history of recently being restored within the past few days to few months. A complaint by a patient will be a first-time complaint, and the sensitivity is more often to air, cold, or food and less likely to heat. The patient's symptoms will resolve quickly after the stimulus is removed, and the tooth will have no radiographic changes.

A patient with irreversible pulpitis will have a history of spontaneous pain with lingering and/or severe pain; after the removal of the stimulus, the pain in many cases continues. Patients feel they know which tooth is bothering them, and the pain tends to increase in duration and frequency over time. Often, you can see radiographic evidence of periapical issues. In a necrotic pulp, the signs and symptoms are similar to irreversible pulpitis. The pain is spontaneous and can be diffuse throughout the dental arch, and radiographic evidence or periapical lesion may or may not be present. You may also see a draining fistula in the area so look around.

When evaluating the radiograph for radiolucent or radiopaque areas, you should consider the following diagnosis.

RADIOLUCENT LESIONS

- **Ameloblastoma** occurs in both arches, are unilocular or multilocular in appearance, and aggressive but benign. Patients are usually symptom-free, teeth respond as normal to pulp testing, and expansion of bone and destruction of tooth and bone are possible.
- **Ameloblastic fibroma** usually occurs in younger patients, is located in a posterior mandible, and can be unilocular or multilocular. The pulp tests normally. Ameloblastic fibromas are benign and slow growing.
- **Central giant-cell granuloma** is usually located around mandibular premolars and anterior teeth in younger patients. It can be unilocular or multilocular, is aggressive in nature, and can destroy bone and cause teeth to move.

- A **dentigerous cyst** usually occurs around unerupted or impacted third molars and maxillary canines. It tends to occur in younger patients, is unilocular in appearance, and is destructive in nature, causing resorption. The teeth test normal to pulp testing.
- A **globulomaxillary cyst** usually occurs between the maxillary canine and lateral incisor, is usually unilocular in shape, and is not destructive. The patient is symptom-free, and teeth test normal to pulp testing.
- A **keratocyst** usually occurs in the mandibular posterior region. It can be unilocular or multilocular in shape with high frequency to reoccur. Pulp test is normal, but you may see bone and tooth resorption.
- A **lateral periodontal cyst** is usually located in mandibular canines and premolar areas. It can be unilocular or multilocular in appearance. Teeth respond normally to pulp testing, and patients are symptom-free.
- A **median palatal cyst** occurs in the midline region of the maxilla posterior to anterior teeth. It is usually unilocular in shape, seen in adults, and responds normally to pulp testing. Patients are free from symptoms except swelling.
- A **nasopalatine duct cyst** occurs between the maxillary central incisors. It is unilocular in shape. Pulp responds normally to pulp testing, and no symptoms are present.
- A **primordial cyst** occurs anywhere but most commonly after a tooth has been extracted. It can be found at any age, and no symptoms are present.
- A **residual cyst** occurs anywhere, is usually unilocular, and doesn't increase in size. There are no symptoms, and the pulp test is normal.
- **Scar tissue** occurs from previous pulpal irritation. It can occur in either arch at any age, and it won't resolve even after root-canal treatment.
- A **traumatic bone cyst** usually occurs in a mandible. Pulp tests normal, and there are no symptoms. It usually occurs in younger patients and may have a scalloped border in appearance.

RADIOPAQUE LESIONS

- **Cementoma**, most common in middle-aged African American females, is usually located in the anterior mandible region. All teeth respond to pulp testing, and the patient is symptom-free.
- **Condensing osteitis** occurs in all ages. It is a reaction of periradicular bone to chronic inflammation of pulp. It can occur anywhere but mostly in the mandibular molar and premolar regions. The patient is symptom-free, and teeth respond to pulp testing.
- **Fibrous dysplasia** occurs in younger patients, is slow growing, and more frequent in the maxilla. The patient is symptom-free, and lesions have the appearance of ground glass.
- **Odontoma** occurs in all patient groups. The radiopacity is made up of enamel dentin and cementum. The patient is symptom-free.
- **Ossifying fibroma** is more common in young adults. It can be found anywhere but is more common in the posterior mandible. It is slow growing. Patients are symptom-free; however, you will sometimes see expansion of bone and displacement of teeth.

- **Osteoblastoma** is usually seen in the mandible posterior region in younger patients. It can cause resorption of tooth structure and expansion of bone with a radiolucent border around the lesion.
- **Osteosarcoma**, a true malignant tumor, usually occurs in younger patients and more commonly in the mandible than maxilla. The patient will commonly have pain, and the tumor has a sunburst appearance.

INSTRUMENTS IN NONSURGICAL ROOT-CANAL PROCEDURES

Consider the following basic setup:

- Rubber dam,
- Rubber dam frame,
- Rubber dam clamp,
- Burs, such as size two, four, and six round,
- Long shank 556,
- Safe-ended diamonds such as endo bur,
- Root-canal broach,
- Rotary orifice shaping instruments,
- Sodium hypochlorite irrigating solutions,
- EDTA or ethylenediaminetetraacetic acid, and
- Root-canal files (either K-files to shape and clean in a push-pull manner, Hedstrom files, which work more in a scraping motion, or reamers, which cut less and are less aggressive).

Remember that files are generally manufactured in lengths ranging from twenty-one to thirty-one millimeters and have a standard taper of point-zero-two-millimeter increase per millimeter increase in length. A size-twenty-five instrument means the apical dimension is point two five millimeters at the apex and increases in diameter point zero two millimeters every additional millimeter in length. You also will need obturation materials and sealers in your setup.

The next steps in your root-canal procedure will be finding your working length and then cleaning and shaping the root canal. Working distance can be defined as the distance from a reproducible point on the coronal portion of the tooth to an identifiable point in the apical portion of the root. Remember, the apical foramen usually exits from the canal anywhere from point five to two millimeters more coronally than how it appears on the radiograph. Once your working distance has been determined, the following steps—cleaning, shaping, and disinfection—are perhaps the most important. Consider the crown-down technique, which means cleaning the coronal two-thirds to three-fourths of the canal to remove the bulk of necrotic tissue and then working the remainder of the canal to the apex.

In the event of a perforation, which can and will happen to all dentists, first review its location. Is it located at the top, middle, or lower third of the tooth? If located in the upper third, will crown lengthening allow you to continue to save the tooth? I recommend that you inform before you perform any procedure, but this is particularly true with root-canal procedures. If you feel the tooth has a good long-term prognosis, then the following steps are in order. First, prevent contamination as much as possible; second, control hemorrhaging with a sterile cotton pellet and pressure; and third, seal immediately with MTA and cover the area with glass ionomer. Complete your root-canal procedure, document the event in your clinical notes, and follow up with appropriate radiographs in three months, six months, and then annually after that.

Here are some tips for dealing with endodontic emergencies. One major problem can be getting your patient comfortable with local anesthesia. You may want to consider a Gow-Gates injection, developed by Dr. G. Gow-Gates in 1973, which is helpful with mandibular nerve-block problems. The technique requires the insertion of a needle, usually a twenty-seven-gauge, more superior and more lateral with respect to the ramus. You must bury the entire length of the needle within the soft tissue. Aspirate often to make sure you have avoided any blood vessels. Other options to consider include a periodontal ligament injection, an intraosseous injection, or an intrapulpal injection.

Another area that needs to be addressed is treatment of traumatic tooth injuries, which is well-documented by the American Association of Endodontists and by Andreasen and Andreasen in the *Textbook and Color Atlas of Traumatic Injuries to the Teeth*, fourth edition. You should first identify whether the injury is acute (the injury occurred within the past few hours), subacute (occurrence within the first twenty-four hours of surgery), or delayed (more than one day old). Next, you should identify whether the injury is a concussion, subluxation, extrusion, lateral luxation, intrusion, or some combination. The next diagnostic decision is to determine what you are dealing with. A primary tooth or a permanent tooth? Is the apex of the tooth completely formed or still developing?

Let's start with treatment guidelines for luxated teeth that are permanent with an apex that is fully formed. With a tooth concussion, the tooth is tender to touch but harbors no displacement or mobility issues, and the radiograph is normal. Consider a flexible splint, if necessary, for seven to ten days. With subluxation, the tooth is tender to touch and mobile, with slight bleeding around the cervical crevice but a normal radiograph. Consider a flexible splint, if necessary or for the patient's comfort, for seven to ten days. With extrusion, the tooth appears elongated and mobile, and radiographic images will show a widened periodontal space. Treatment will consist of repositioning and stabilizing the tooth with a flexible splint for about three months.

With lateral luxation, a tooth is displaced axially and usually locked into the bone, but it is not tender to touch or mobile. It appears almost ankylotic, and the radiograph will show a widened periodontal ligament. Treatment requires repositioning the tooth, and in most cases a local anesthetic will be necessary, as well as placement of a flexible splint for three to six weeks. With intrusion, a tooth is displaced deeper into the alveolar bone, is not tender to touch, and not mobile. The radiograph is inconclusive. Treat by repositioning the tooth and, if the apex is fully formed, providing root-canal treatment within one to three weeks. In all of these cases, consider recommending use of a soft toothbrush after each meal along with a chlorhexidine mouth rinse of .12 percent twice a day for two weeks. In most cases, teeth with extrusive and lateral and intrusive luxation injuries will need root-canal treatment.

Treatment for avulsed permanent teeth with closed apex can be reviewed under three categories:

1. When the tooth has already been replanted
2. When the tooth has been kept in a special storage medium and extraoral drying time is less than sixty minutes
3. When the tooth has been out of the mouth and exposed to drying greater than sixty minutes.

In the first situation, clean the area with chlorhexidine and do not extract. Suture the gingiva if necessary, radiograph the area, administer systemic antibiotics, and consider a tetanus booster if the avulsed tooth has been exposed to soil or if tetanus coverage is uncertain.

When the second issue occurs, clean the root surface with sterile saline, remove the coagulum from the socket area with sterile saline, and slowly reimplant, providing systemic antibiotics.

When the third issue occurs, you should remove the debris on the tooth and coagulum from the socket with sterile saline, immerse the tooth for five minutes in sodium fluoride, and then reimplant slowly into the socket, providing systemic antibiotics.

In all of the above treatments, home-care instructions should include a soft diet for two weeks, brushing after each meal with a soft toothbrush, and use of chlorhexidine mouth rinse .12 percent twice a day for one week. In most cases, you should consider root-canal treatment within two weeks.

Treatment for avulsed permanent teeth with an open apex is the same as with a closed apex, except in the following manner. When the tooth has been exposed to drying for less than sixty minutes, consider soaking the tooth in doxycycline, a concentration of one hundred milligrams of doxycycline in twenty milliliters of sterile saline, for one to two minutes before implanting. If the tooth has been exposed to drying for longer than sixty minutes, replantation is usually not indicated. In the above cases, consider root-canal care with calcium hydroxide to encourage apexification and obturate with gutta-percha. Follow up with radiographs at three, six, and twelve months. Prognosis is based on the amount of time the tooth was out of the mouth, but in all cases the prognosis will be poor.

When dealing with tooth fractures, you must consider the location of the fracture and if it is vertical or horizontal. The classifications are apical third, middle third, and coronal third. In the apical third, the tooth should be repositioned and splinted for six to eight weeks; usually, root-canal care will be unnecessary. When the fracture occurs in the middle third, reposition the coronal portion, place a rigid splint for six to eight weeks, and provide root-canal procedures only in the coronal portion of the tooth. When the fracture occurs in the coronal third, it is usually the most difficult to treat. Reposition the tooth and place a rigid splint for six to eight weeks (which may be very difficult to do, and often the coronal portion of the tooth will be lost). In many cases, the tooth may need to be orthodontically extruded. If you attempt to save or simply remove the tooth, consider prosthetic options.

RESORPTION ISSUES

We first deal with internal resorption that is nonperforated; you will treat this like any other root-canal procedure and likely will have a success rate similar to routine root-canal procedures (about 85–95 percent success). When you encounter internal resorption that has perforation, treatment should occur within days of your diagnosis, and the prognosis is much poorer. In these cases, use a calcium hydroxide and barium sulfate mix as a hemostatic agent in a ratio of six to one. This helps you find the perforation and determine the size of the defect, since in many cases it will not always be evident. You will need copious amounts of 6 percent sodium hypochlorite to irrigate the canal or canals while cleaning and shaping them. If hemorrhage is an issue, you may need to leave the sodium hypochlorite in the canal for several minutes. If hemorrhage continues to be an issue, you may want to consider packing the canal with calcium hydroxide for seven to fourteen days and, in some cases, a surgical approach will be necessary to remove the external granulation tissue before obturation of the canal. The treatment approach for external root resorption is the same as for internal resorption that has perforated. In most cases, external resorption will be associated with some type of avulsion injury.

APEXOGENESIS AND APEXIFICATION

Apexogenesis is a biological process that occurs in teeth with incomplete apical formation, where the pulp tissue is protected and encouraged to allow the process of normal root development and apical closure. Apexification occurs in teeth with necrotic pulps and occurs when root-canal treatment has occurred, and filling and sealing material allows a hard tissue barrier to form.

In both cases, you will clean and shape the canal with sodium hypochlorite solution and use either calcium hydroxide as filler for six months or permanent MTA (mineral trioxide aggregate). Placing either material can be a challenge so consider the use of NiTi files, pluggers, rotary compactors, or injectable types of products. Remember, the most common reason for failure is inadequate coronal seal. Make sure your technique for bonding is spot-on for the composite restoration.

DENTAL PULP AND PERIODONTAL INTERACTION

Can one disease cause or interact with the other? Who cares! In many cases, you will need to treat both issues together for the best prognosis. The problem can be classified as primary pulpal disease, primary pulpal disease with secondary periodontal disease, primary periodontal disease, primary periodontal disease with secondary pulpal disease, combined pulpal and periodontal disease, or concomitant pulpal and periodontal disease. Before you start treatment, review long-term prognoses and cost factors, realizing that in many cases both will need to be treated together for best results. Often, broad-based periodontal probing will be associated with periodontal disease and narrow-based probing will be associated with endodontic lesions.

CRACKED TOOTH SYNDROME

First, look for craze lines, fractured cusps, large undermining amalgams, intraradicular posts or pins, unrestored endodontically treated teeth, traumatic occlusion, and tooth abrasion and erosion. Subjective finding can also be very helpful. The most pathognomonic sign for a cracked tooth is pain upon mastication; however, upon release of force the pain goes away. This sign only occurs in vital teeth, never in endodontically treated teeth or necrotic teeth.

RESTORING ENDODONTICALLY TREATED TEETH

Remember, posts only hold the restorative core portion in place; they do not give strength to a tooth. Reasons for not using posts often include having to remove additional sound tooth structure, as posts offer no additional strength and can increase the chance of root fracture. If a post must be used, remember that it should not be greater than one-third of the entire root width in all directions. Try to resist placing posts in mesial roots of mandibular molars and buccal roots of maxillary molars; also, avoid large posts in the distal roots of mandibular molars and palatal roots of maxillary molars if possible.

In the end, the best advice I can give is to call your patient the evening of the surgery to see how he or she is doing. Inform your patient before you perform. Make sure your patient understands that 5–15 percent of all root canals fail no matter what you do. Make sure he or she understands that in most cases, a buildup and crown will be needed after root-canal treatment, and additional costs will be incurred. Please also inform patients that postendodontic signs and symptoms may persist for some time so be patient.

11. ORAL SURGERY

THE BEST WAY to start oral surgical procedures (and perhaps any medical or dental care) is with a review of the patient's past and present medical and dental history, along with recording their chief complaint. You should review any current and past medications, any history of allergies, and the need for preoperative antibiotics, as well as the need for a medical consultation when appropriate, blood work, and review of blood-sugar levels. I suggest a complete clinical exam, including restorative charting of what has been done and what needs to be done and periodontal charting. I recommend documenting ranges of motion vertically and laterally, protrusive of the lower jaw, and any clicking, popping, or crepitus in either the right or left TMJ, along with any deflections or deviations upon opening and/or closing of the lower jaw. Make sure you have all preoperative radiographs necessary for treatment. Next, all vital signs should be documented: blood pressure, heartrate, respiration rate, and temperature. All informed consents should be signed and reviewed. Again, inform before you perform.

Surgical instrumentation will vary depending on procedure and operator preference. However, a basic setup should include the following:

- Syringe
- Needle
- Local anesthetic
- Hemostat curved
- Blade handle
- Dissecting scissors curved
- Straight elevator
- Crane pick
- Needle holder
- Sterile gauze four-by-four
- Periosteal elevator
- Double-ended curette and bone file
- Retractors
- Sutures size two cutting a three-eighths circle twenty-four millimeters
- Surgical hand piece

- Burs
- Mouth props

The most common procedure will be extractions, especially third-molar removals. Classification of impactions are vertical, horizontal, mesioangular, and distoangular, and they can be either tissue covered, bony covered, or a combination. Remember that for insurance purposes, the classification can have a large impact on fees received.

Here is a summary of surgical tips for removing mandibular third molars, starting with vertical impactions. Step one is flap design, which should be done with a size-fifteen blade, and the first incision is from distal of the second molar along the external oblique ridge toward the ascending ramus for about one inch. The second incision is made from the distal of the second molar, extending in a vertical direction toward the mucobuccal fold for about one inch. Remember, the incision goes down to bone and the second incision should go beyond the mucogingival junction. When opening the flap, remember to do a full thickness flap, lifting the periosteum. You should then focus on bone removal, exposing the crown of the impacted tooth with a size-eight surgical round bur. Then, create a purchase point in the crown and use your crane pick in an up-and-down motion to loosen the tooth. Once the tooth has been removed, the socket is flushed with clean water and the flap replaced and sutured with two-zero gut. Home-care instructions are given.

The technique with mesioangular lower impactions is as follows. The flap design is the same; however, in this case you should consider using your size-eight round surgical bur, making a vertical groove through the crown but stopping short of cutting right through the lingual portion of the crown for fear of nerve damage. Then, use a number-one C gouge elevator and place the tooth into mesial and distal portions of the groove that was just cut and split. Then continue with the number-one C and remove the distal portion of the tooth first, proceeding to remove the mesial portion with a number-eight crane pick. Clean and close as described above.

For horizontal impactions, flap design is the same; however, you should use your size-eight round bur and cut through the crown at the cementoenamel junction. Go through almost the entire crown but stop short of breaking through the lingual. You then use the number-one C gouge elevator to separate the crown from the root structure, removing the crown portion of the tooth first. Then, create a purchase point in the remaining root structure. Use your crane pick to remove the root portion and then clean and close the wound area as described above.

When removing a distoangular impaction, use the same flap design as described above. Then use the size-eight round bur to section the tooth at the cementoenamel junction, almost through to the lingual but again stop short. Then use the number-one C gouge elevator to section the crown from the root, making sure you have freed the bone from the ascending ramus so the crown portion can be removed. A purchase point is then made into the remaining root structure, and the crane pick is used to remove the remaining root structure. The area is then cleaned and closed as described above.

Here are some surgical tips for removing maxillary impacted teeth. First, the classification is the same, along with the technique, for all types of maxillary impactions. The first step is flap design, and the first incision is from the distal of the second molar along the tuberosity midcrestal down to bone, about one inch long. The second incision starts at the mesial of the second molar, in a vertical fashion toward and then past the mucogingival junction, also down to bone. A full thickness flap is raised with a number sixty-nine periosteal elevator. The next step is to use a chisel or surgical size-eight round burs to remove the buccal bone and expose the crown portion of the impacted tooth. The number-one C gouge is then placed on the mesial surface of the crown and adjacent bone, and with leverage, the tooth is luxated out. The wound is then cleaned and closed the same way as mandibular impactions.

These steps are for the surgical removal of erupted mandibular molars. Start with an intrasulcular incision with two vertically releasing incisions past the MGJ at the line angles of adjacent teeth. Then, section the mesial and distal portions of the tooth so that you have divided the tooth into mesial and distal halves and remove each section with your east-west elevators. Clean and close as described earlier.

A summary of the surgical removal of erupted maxillary molars is as follows. A flap is created intrasulcular with one or two vertically releasing incisions past the MGJ, and the full flap is raised. Remember, the vertically releasing incision starts at the adjacent teeth-line angle. You must then section the tooth vertically, separating the palatal aspect from the buccal aspect. A second groove with round eight is then done, separating the mesial from the distal root structure. Then, remove the mesial and distal roots and then the palatal roots. Clean and close as previously described.

FRENECTOMIES

In most cases, you will be doing a maxillary labial frenectomy for preprosthetic reasons, creating room for an upper denture or helping to eliminate a diastema. In the mandibular area, you will be removing the lingual frenum in cases of ankyloglossia.

The following steps should be taken to remove the maxillary labial frenum for preprosthetic reasons. Take a small curved hemostat and grab the frenum about three-fourths of an inch above the crestal attachment, where it inserts into the upper lip. The hemostat is held at a ninety-degree angle to the labial surface. Then, take your scissors, which are held at approximately ninety degrees to the ridge, and cut. The scissors should be in front of the hemostat, toward the crest of the ridge. After that initial cut, you then take your scissors and hold them parallel to the crest of the ridge. Starting at the crest of the ridge, remove the entire frenum. The area should be sutured with two-gut suture.

Removal of the maxillary frenum to help close a diastema is very similar but utilizes a slightly different technique. The frenectomy is indicated when the frenum goes completely through the diastema and attaches into the incisive papilla, and, when stretched or tugged on, the tissue blanches. Grab the frenum with your curved hemostat under the upper lip, use scissors to cut above your hemostat toward the upper lip, and make that initial cut to bone.

Then use your size-fifteen blade to make two additional incisions down to the bone on the mesial and distal of the frenum up to the crest of the ridge so that the entire maxillary frenum can be removed. Next, take a diamond or fissure bur and cut a groove between teeth eight and nine, scoring the periosteum. A circular cut is then made to remove the incisive papilla up through the diastema. The bleeding can be controlled with Acu-Surg, laser, or similar device and/or a two-gut suture.

The lingual frenectomy is done when the movement of the tongue is restricted. In many cases when a patient is unable to touch his or her upper lip with the tongue, the frenectomy is indicated. The patient's tongue is held with a four-by-four or suture, pulling it up and out, and a curved hemostat is used to grab the frenum where it attaches to the ventral surface of the tongue. Then take your scissors and, above the hemostat and parallel to the hemostat, make your first cut toward the tongue. The area is then sutured with a two- zero gut suture.

DRY SOCKET

The dry socket, or alveolar osteitis, is very painful and a common postoperative complication. In most cases, you will find it occurs more on the lower arch. First, local anesthesia must be given. Then clean or debride the socket out with a curette, right down to the base of the extraction site. Then, consider a fifty-fifty mix of saline and hydrogen peroxide to flush the area out three to four times. If any necrotic bone is present, you should remove it. Pack the extraction site with Dressol-X; start at the base of the socket so all walls of the extraction site are covered. You should then remove the packing in three to seven days; in some cases, this will need to be done two to three times.

Perhaps the most important aspect to remember in contemplating all procedures is inform before you perform. Call your patient in the evening to make sure there are no postoperative complications. I also suggest preoperative pain medication the day before and morning of the event and antibiotics when indicated.

12. RESTORATIONS

At this point, I will speak about amalgams and composites. Let us first talk about amalgams. In most contemporary practices, the discussion of amalgams will be short. However, in my opinion there is still a place for their use in most dental practices. In an ideal world, we often could avoid their use, but in the real world, you may want to consider them. When gingival tissue will be in the way, and the patient, for whatever reason, is unable or unwilling to have his or her soft tissue recontoured, and moisture control and a rubber dam are unable to be placed, I think you should consider the amalgam restoration as an option. Composite restorations will not hold up as well as an amalgam when placed in a wet or moist surgical field. Second and third molars, where access is usually difficult, are other areas for amalgam use.

With over thirty clinical years of practicing general dentistry and often working with new dental-school graduates, I've learned that the difficult part of doing general dentistry is performing a composite restoration that looks good, functions and wears well, has nice interproximal contacts, and is not sensitive. I am very aware of how the public wants and demands, in many cases, the tooth colored or composite restoration. However, the delivery of that restoration creates more clinical problems than anything else we do in our organization. In my opinion, the number-one reason for such problems is poor patient selection and treatment plan. In most cases, a much better treatment plan would be an inlay, onlay, or crown rather than a very large and complex composite restoration.

When the patient refuses the correct treatment plan, please consider having him or her sign a noncompliance form. Such form must be signed by the doctor and the patient, stating what you have recommended for treatment and what your patient has elected to do. I am very aware that performing treatment you do not agree with should be avoided. However, in the real world, often you will make compromises. You may be well-intentioned, but you will have problems. The noncompliance form decreases the chances of an average patient requesting that failing treatment be done at no charge or the patient taking actions against you or your company for the care not holding up. My personal feelings are that composites should not be done on second or third molars, on teeth that will require more than three surfaces, or when more than one-third of the occlusal surface will need to be restored. I recommend informing all patients scheduling large restorations that you expect them to have sensitivity and, if that continues, root-canal treatment, and most likely a crown will be needed. This statement should be made before you perform, not after. When stated before treatment, you appear as an astute clinician; when done afterward, you appear to be making an excuse. I also suggest that on all posterior composites, you have your patient sign an informed consent stating that the fees for composites tend to be higher and that out-of-pocket expenses may be greater. In most cases, I inform the patient that insurance companies will sometimes consider composites cosmetic in nature, but with anterior teeth that is not the situation.

13. Orthodontics

In 75–80 percent of orthodontic cases, lack of space is the issue and crowding becomes the patient's primary concern. The next most important concern is that teeth are too protrusive. As you look at your patient, I recommend that you fully understand his or her primary compliant. I then suggest that your diagnosis determine if the problem is coming from the skeletal upper arch, skeletal lower arch, a clockwise or counterclockwise grower, the upper teeth position or lower teeth position, or some combination of all. The next issue is determining whether treatment should begin right away or if it can be postponed until the patient is older. If your diagnosis leads you to a growth issue and the patient is compliant, you should start care and treatment early. If the problem is just going to require leveling, alignment, and rotation, then treatment can be started almost any time.

The best way to make a determination is through complete orthodontic records. Records should have a cephalometric, panoramic, and full-mouth series of radiographs. You should also have upper and lower impressions along with a centric occlusal bite, intra- and extraoral photos with the intraoral photos being of upper and lower teeth two to four millimeters apart, upper and lower anterior teeth together, natural smile to determine the amount of gingiva present, right and left cuspid, and upper and lower occlusal views. For extraoral views, I suggest right and left profile views and straight-on views with and without a smile. I also suggest an orthodontic exam of the right and left TMJ, checking for popping, clicking, crepitus, deflections, and/or deviation as well as any pain on loading the right and left TMJ.

I recommend you evaluate the patient's airway to determine whether he or she is a mouth breather, nasal breather, or a combination of both. You should evaluate the periodontal condition, in particular any areas of lack of attached gingiva, along with the amount of crowding or spacing present in both arches. I also suggest you evaluate the patient's face: is it pleasing to look at? Are the lips full or thin; is the chin protrusive or retrusive; does the patient show a lot of his or her maxillary gingiva or very little? I suggest a tracing of the patient's cephalometric film be completed based on sex, age, and race. I suggest, too, that you charge a fee for the orthodontic records. Whether you apply that fee to the accepted treatment or not is an individual decision. I personally charge a fee for records and consultation, and if the patient elects to go forward, I apply that fee toward his or her orthodontic care.

Since crowding is the most common problem, I start with the two most common methods of gaining space: extraction of teeth and/or expansion, meaning we will move posterior teeth backward and/or possibly move molars laterally. In a best possible situation, we would avoid orthodontic problems altogether with early diagnoses and treatment. How can we reduce or eliminate them? In most cases, enlarged tonsils, airway problems, and thumb, finger, and tongue habits are the cause. Your orthodontic records, along with clinical experience, should allow you to answer the following questions before you attempt care and treatment. First, is treatment necessary? Second, how should space be gained to move teeth? Third, what does the cephalometric diagnosis tell us about where the teeth and/or jaw relationship should be placed? Fourth, what tooth movements will be necessary to accomplish treatment? Finally, what is the prognosis of your care and treatment?

Consider the following orthodontic problems and treatment options.

Example 1: Crowded anterior teeth with good jaw relationship. When crowding is more than five to six millimeters, consider extraction of the first premolars on upper and lower arches. Then retract the canines to make room to align and level the upper and lower anterior teeth. Then move the molars mesial into any remaining space.

Example 2: Maxillary arch is protrusive and lower arch is fine. One option is to move the maxillary molars distally, retract the premolars and canines, and then retract the upper anterior. The second option is to extract the maxillary first premolars, retract the canines, and then retract the anterior teeth.

Example 3: Bimaxillary protrusion, meaning the lips and midface are too full. Consider extraction of both upper and lower first premolars and then retract the canines, followed by the anterior teeth. Keep in mind that generally, whenever you perform extractions of premolars, you tend to increase or deepen the bite, meaning greater overbite, and that when you distalize or expand, you tend to open the bite. Understanding this concept will guide you when you are not sure which procedure to consider—extraction or expansion. If the patient has an open bite, you may want to lean toward extraction; if your patient has a deep bite, you may want to consider expansion, all other factors being equal. You must also realize that the amount of expansion or distalization has limitations. Generally, you can distalize upper molars five to seven millimeters; however, on the lower arch you are only able to distalize the molars one to two millimeters. This means that the mandibular arch is the limited arch and tends to dictate care and treatment. If you remove premolars in the lower arch, you usually remove them in the upper arch as well. However, as mentioned earlier, you will often remove maxillary premolars and not need to remove mandibular premolars in cases of maxillary protrusion. We have now decided that the lower arch will guide our treatment. The following options are available for review of the lower arch.

- No crowding and incisors are proclined: consider extraction
- Crowding less than two millimeters/side and no incisor proclination: consider expansion.
- Crowding less than two millimeters/side and incisor proclination: consider expansion.
- Crowding more than two millimeters/side and no incisor proclination: consider extraction.
- Crowding more than two millimeters/side and incisor proclination: consider extraction.

Although this seems very straightforward, you must determine which stage of the dentition you are dealing with, such as primary, mixed, or permanent. The transition from mixed to permanent becomes important in reviewing the term "leeway space." The primary cuspid is one millimeter less in mesial distal width than the permanent cuspid. First primary molars are one millimeter wider mesial distally than permanent first premolars. Second primary molars are two and a half millimeters wider mesial distally than permanent second premolars. This space difference means we can get another two and a half millimeters per side on the lower arch, or a total of five millimeters to relieve crowding on the lower arch if we can prevent the permanent lower first molar from drifting mesial. This is mostly done by placing a lower lingual arch.

The art of orthodontic care comes from deciding what to do when we need to extract but do not want to close the bite or, conversely, we want to expand but do not want to open the bite. This will force you to look at your patient's facial growth pattern. If the patient is a clockwise grower, he or she will have a strong tendency to have an open bite; if your patient has a tendency to be a counterclockwise grower, he or she will have a tendency to have a deep bite. In these cases, compromise may be necessary. In general, for a patient for whom you want to open the bite but who is a counterclockwise grower, you may want to consider expansion. Conversely, when you want to close a patient's bite but he or she is a clockwise grower, you may want to consider extractions. Such growth patterns tend to provide certain profiles; for example, the prognathic profile, or large-chin deep biters, tends to be a counterclockwise grower, while small-chin open biters tend to be clockwise growers or retrognathic in appearance.

You should have a good idea now where you will be considering extractions, expansion, or neither. The next question concerns how you move the teeth. Remember, every action will have a reaction force so the goal is to control tooth movements. In basic terms, you must understand anchorage, which can be minimal, moderate, or maximal. In the example of the extraction of the first premolar, a space has been created, and now you have to decide whether you want to move the anterior and posterior segments equally toward one another, move the anterior segment more than the posterior segment, or move the posterior segment more than the anterior segment. This is where anchorage will come into play.

While we are on the subject, remember that two movements need to occur when moving teeth. First, the crown has to move. This occurs very quickly and easily, and it is called tipping. However, the second movement is the root movement into proper position; this is called torque, and it takes much longer.

We should now talk about the three common force systems used to move teeth. Class one force, or intra-arch force, entails one system; a good example is retracting cuspid to molar in the same arch. For class two force, a good example is retracting the maxillary cuspid by placing a force from mandibular molars to the maxillary cuspid so that you are correcting class two problems by retraction of the maxillary segment and protraction of the mandibular posterior segment. The class-three segment is another type of interarch system in which you correct class-three problems by retracting the mandibular anterior segment and protracting the maxillary posterior segment.

When deciding on whether orthodontic treatment should be done, ask yourself the following questions:

- Are the cuspid and first molars in class one occlusion?
- Are the overbite and overjet within normal limits? Usually those would be one to three millimeters vertically and horizontally.
- Are all spaces closed, and is no crowding present?
- Are the lips, nose, and chin in balance? Normally the lower lip will be one to two millimeters behind the esthetic plane, which is a line from the tip of the nose to the tip of the chin.
- Is the TMJ comfortable, and the range of motion within normal limits?

If the answers to these questions are all yes, then in many cases orthodontic care may not be necessary clinically. Still, many patients will seek care and treatment.

Some discussion at this point about Invisalign devices is appropriate. In general, many patients are interested in Invisalign, and I have been providing this kind of care for almost fifteen years. First, remember that you need excellent patient compliance. If the aligners are not worn, treatment will not be successful. In general, I do not strongly recommend Invisalign to younger patients because of the high probability of lost aligners. However, keep in mind that patients with less than ideal hygiene will often do better with Invisalign than conventional bands and brackets. Although excellent results can be achieved with Invisalign, I find that skeletal and tooth rotation issues can be much slower in moving teeth, and it's harder to predict final tooth position.

It is very important that excellent and accurate impressions be taken and all other orthodontic records be done. If the impressions are not clear, you are wasting time and money. Just redo those impressions before you dismiss your patient, or he or she will just end up coming back. Actually, I suggest two sets of impressions, decreasing the need to have patients return for new impressions. Remember, patients should not eat or drink with these retainers in their mouth, and they should strive to wear them for sixteen to twenty hours a day. The aligners should be changed every two weeks, and most crowding will be resolved with air rotor slenderizing (ARS).

Some discussion should also take place regarding fixed versus removable appliances. In my opinion, unless you have specific reasons, focus should be on fixed appliances since patient cooperation can be a challenge. If your patient has jaw issues and is still in the growth phase, be aware of what functional appliances can accomplish if they are constructed properly and worn consistently. Excellent results can be achieved. However, these days it will be an uphill battle. Remember not to promise the world; instead, I suggest underpromising and overdelivering. The same can be stated for headgear. Headgear may be the appliance of choice; however, patient cooperation is tricky. Even though it may be the correct treatment choice, understand that young children often will not be compliant.

Most orthodontic emergencies will involve a wire cutting a cheek or a band or bracket coming off. You should be familiar with an orthodontic end cutter to cut long wires. You should know how to tie in an arch wire and rebracket loose brackets. Keep in mind that if you center the bracket onto the tooth, with the bracket slot in the middle of the tooth, or from incisal edge, to free-gingival margin and the midpoint from mesial to distal, you will be safe in most instances. Remember, the tapered or narrow end of the bracket goes toward the gingiva, and the closer the bracket is placed toward the gingiva the more you will extrude the tooth. The more you place the bracket toward the incisal edge, the more you will intrude the tooth. In most cases, you will be dealing with straight wire orthodontics, meaning the tip and torque is built into the bracket. The patient will have nickel-titanium wires going from round wire 012, 014, 016, 018, and 020 to 016 by 022 rectangular wires. In most cases, a patient will need to be seen every six to eight weeks, and in most cases, treatment will take at least eighteen to twenty-four months.

The round wire will allow for tipping, aligning, and leveling, and the rectangular wire will allow for torqueing or moving the roots into proper position. I recommend that all patients understand that if they want to keep teeth straight, they must commit to permanent retention, whether fixed or removable. I recommend that upon completion of all orthodontic treatment, complete postorthodontic records are recorded; they should be the same types of records that were taken before you started the orthodontic case.

Orthodontics can be rewarding dentistry and smart business. Most orthodontic treatments do not cause pain. Even when money is tight, most parents will find a way to provide orthodontic care for their children. In most cases, you will incur no accounts receivable, and most orthodontics can be delegated out to support staff. Although this chapter's goal is not to have practices initiate orthodontic care, I do suggest consideration of appropriate training to improve knowledge, and I recommend the seminars of the International Association for Orthodontics (IAO) and the Progressive Orthodontic Seminars (POS).

14. IMPLANTOLOGY

As BEFORE, AN overview of implantology starts with complete patient records. These include past medical and dental history, charting of existing restorations and restorations needed, complete periodontal charting, impressions of and bite of upper and lower arches, diagnostic intra- and extraoral photos, Panorex, a CAT scan when indicated, and periapical radiographs. After evaluating the radiographs, you should be able to document the shape of the upper and lower jaws as A, B, C, D, or E (from best to worst, with the A and B having the most height and width). You can also document the quality of bone as category one, two, three, or four (again, from best to worst, with one and two having the most cortical or dense bone). In most cases, your ideal cases will have a shape of A or B and a quality of one or two. If your patient selection falls into those categories, you will have many successful cases.

Next, consider your patient's chief complaint and then check the condition of surrounding teeth. If the abutment teeth are in excellent condition, all things being equal, I suggest you guide the patient toward implant treatment. If the condition of such teeth is poor, with existing restorations, I suggest conventional crown-and-bridge treatment.

An additional condition that should be examined but is often missed in treatment planning of dental implants is interocclusal space. In other words, will you have enough room after the implant is placed to do your prosthesis, and will you have enough abutment height to retain a cemented restoration? If not, you may need to take steps to create appropriate space or compromise with a screw-retained restoration rather than a cemented one. Please keep in mind, this review would only take care of retention and may not provide the ideal shape and contour of a future restoration.

The next area to review is the height and width of bone, along with quality of bone and the amount and type of tissue available. Will enough attached gingiva be present? Will presurgical care be necessary? For most of you reviewing this section, you only will be concerned with cylinder-type implants. However, you should be aware of options such as blade implants and subperiosteal implants. Blade-type implants will often be an option in the posterior mandible with narrow ridges. The typical blade implant will be one point two to one point eight millimeters wide and can be tied into the natural dentition. Subperiosteal implants are, in most cases, treatment planned for the edentulous patient, ones where you do not have enough bone to place the implant. In these types of situations, the implant sits on top of the bone. In the end, you will need to address the following factors to make sure you achieve osteointegration and long-term implant success: the biocompatibility and design of the implant, along with surface conditions of the implant; the quality and quantity of the patient's bone; surgical technique; and loading conditions after implant insertion. These factors will determine success or failure.

Implant treatment planning can be reviewed based on patient conditions. Let us start with the fully edentulous patient. You should consider mini-implants, between two to four with O-rings, for patients who may be medically compromised or financially compromised. You should consider conventional implants, meaning a diameter of at least three and a half millimeters. Between two to six implants are usually needed. In most cases, such implants will be placed on the lower arch between mental foramen on the patients left side and mental foramen on the patients right side and on the upper arch between first premolars. When dealing with the edentulous arch on the maxilla, please be aware of the maxillary sinus areas; on the mandible, be aware of the mandibular canal area. Often it is best to avoid these areas by one to two millimeters. When that is not possible, consider sinus lift procedures, tilted implants on the upper arch and on the lower arch, bone grafts, or mandibular nerve relocation. You should know that in most cases, at least two millimeters of space between each implant is recommended for better cleaning and hygiene.

Remember, the prosthesis drives the treatment plan. Is your patient looking for something cemented, screwed down, or snapped on? What drives the decision is how much interocclusal space needs to be taken up by the prosthesis; in other words, how much soft tissue will need to be replaced in the prosthesis, and how long will the teeth need to be? After doing implants for more than thirty years, I feel fixed, detachable prostheses offer the best of all possible worlds. When in place, they are very stable and secure; however, if a problem occurs, and it always will, removal and maintenance will become a lifesaver. Although screw-down types of prostheses meet such a definition, patients are unable to remove them themselves, so when removal is necessary, it can be time-consuming to remove, clean, and place the prosthesis back into your patient's mouth. I believe a treatment plan allowing your patient to remove his or her prosthesis as needed will help avoid many potential issues in the long term.

When treatment planning, you should also evaluate the cantilever action when placing four to six implants in fixed-type prostheses. I suggest avoiding cantilevering any more than twenty millimeters per side, distal to last implant. This should be discussed with your patient prior to treatment, not after. Oftentimes your patient will assume he or she is having second- and third-molar occlusion, and in many cases you may only be providing him or her first-molar or second-premolar occlusion. Such assumptions provide a good time to interject a practice management tip about dental implants. Try not to create a treatment plan for these types of cases à la carte; avoid charging per implant. Simply construct a treatment plan for the case, not the number of implants: a total fee to restore the maxilla or mandible. If you start making a treatment plan for a set number of implants with a fee for each implant and something does not go well, you will be returning funds to patients. A treatment plan with a total fee to restore the edentulous arch is much smarter; it will create fewer problems.

The next type of treatment plan to cover is the replacement of single missing teeth. I suggest considering one implant for each missing tooth. I also recommend you avoid tying natural teeth to implants when considering fixed partial dentures. When considering implants in the anterior section of the mouth from cuspid to cuspid, remember that esthetics should dominate your treatment plan decision. In some cases, unless you are very experienced, I would avoid these areas. Some serious issues include recession and dark triangles between teeth, along with a host of other problems. This situation can best be avoided by appropriate treatment planning before you start the case, not after or during it. Every issue has a solution, but without proper experience and knowledge, mistakes that can be made will be made. Pay close attention and, unless adequately trained, avoid the anterior maxilla with single-type implants unless you have ideal conditions; even when you have them, be very cautious.

Other areas of concern include the height of interproximal bone for proper papilla formation and knowledge of the shape and size of the papilla prior to treatment. When you plan bone-grafting techniques with extractions for future implants, remember to inform patients that if the implant is not placed within six to twelve months, additional grafting will be necessary. Many times, Mr. or Ms. Smith will ask, "Why do I need another graft? I have already had one. Why do I need to pay for another one?" Poor communication with patients enforces the mantra, "Remember, inform before you perform."

Some common questions and answers that should help you in treatment planning are as follows:

- How long will the implant last? I recommend that you consider success to be ten years or greater.
- Does implant surgery hurt? In most cases, implant surgery is less painful than having a tooth removed.
- How long does implant surgery take? In most cases, the placement of a single implant will take less than fifty minutes.
- Do dental implants fail? Yes, about 10 percent fail on the lower arch and 20 percent on the upper arch.

Many factors increase the failure rate, but the most common are smoking, diabetes that is not under control, and poor patient home care. Remember, a dental implant cannot get a cavity, but it can develop periodontal disease. Other common factors include poor quality and quantity of bone and loading or putting the implant into function too soon. In general, I suggest you wait for eight to ten weeks on the lower arch and sixteen to twenty weeks on the upper arch.

Can you place the dental implant immediately after you extract a tooth? Yes, but you have to be able to remove the tooth with as little trauma as possible to provide the implant with the best bone available. I suggest you do not promise your patient that this can be done. If the dental extraction is completed with little to no damage to the surrounding bone, then in many cases, the implant can be placed immediately and good success can be expected.

How much does a dental implant cost? Please make sure your patient understands that at least three different fees may apply. The first fee is the surgical placement of the implant. The second fee is the implant abutment. The third fee is the placement of the implant crown. Your patient should be aware of the total cost before treatment. Remember this!

Maintenance of dental implants should be similar to maintenance of natural teeth. I suggest that radiographs be taken prior to treatment, during surgical procedures and placement of the dental implant, and postoperatively. Radiographs should be taken prior to loading and during impressions to assure abutments are seated correctly, as well as after prostheses are placed. I suggest a follow up with radiographs at six months, twelve months and then every two to three years or as symptoms dictate. Regarding hygiene programs, we suggest scaling with plastic instrumentation and probing as with any natural tooth. Keep in mind that average practitioners probe with a point five to one point five newton centometer of pressure on natural teeth, and I suggest less pressure around implants in order not to break down the soft-tissue seal around the abutments.

In general, mobility of dental implants is usually a sure sign of failure. However, if no pain is present, I suggest you exam the abutment, which in many cases may become loose due to improper torqueing. In most systems, you will need to use a torque wrench and apply thirty to thirty-five nc to make sure your abutment does not come loose. Most practitioners can only hand-tighten to a maximum of ten to fifteen nc. This is very important to understand because if you have cemented your crown over the abutment and the abutment becomes loose, the only way to tighten the abutment is to cut off the crown. This is a waste of money and time, and your patient will not be pleased. Another point to keep in mind is that after tightening the abutment down, make sure you place a cotton pellet in the access hole and then cover that hole with cavit, composite, or Fermit-type material so if you or another practitioner needs access, you will be able to get at it. Please make sure to document in your case notes the type and size of dental implants and their location for future reference. I suggest you provide this information to your patient also. Every day I see a patient having a dental implant issue, and the patient does not know what type of implant was placed or its size—or even when and by whom it was done. This issue will only become more of a problem in time, so please document.

15. Removable Prosthesis

THIS IS AN area often overlooked, but it can offer patients many advantages if done correctly and treatment is planned accordingly. First and most important, under the best of circumstances most patients would prefer something nonremovable. However, due to medical history, financial issues, time, and/or clinical conditions, a removable prosthesis may be a better option for some patients and should be explained and reviewed, along with risks, benefits, alternatives, and costs. In most cases, it is unclear to patients that the removable prosthesis should, and often needs to be, relined periodically and that there is a cost to the procedure. There may be an inconvenience as well since in many cases the patient will have to go without his/her prosthesis while the reline is being completed. Prior to treatment planning, you need complete dental records. As discussed for previous procedures, a review is required of past and current medical history. Include documentation of your patient's chief complaint, a full series of radiographs, Panorex, intra- and extraoral photos, complete dental and periodontal charting, and diagnostic impressions, bite, and mounted cast. Please make sure you review abutment teeth and their condition, as that assessment will often bear the support of your future prosthesis, along with the amount, condition, and adequate attached gingiva. Also, review the amount of bone loss and make sure your patient understands that the use and function of a removable prosthesis will only add to additional bone resorption; with more bone loss, your patient will often need additional adjustment and have more postinsertion difficulties.

The design of your removable prosthesis will start with which type of material should be used, such as acrylic resin, vulcanite, polystyrene, metal, or flexible material. You will then consider clasp type, such as bar, circumferential, rest seats (either incisal, lingual, occlusal), or precision (major connector labial, lingual, or palatal). The guide planes and the height of contour of abutment teeth are other important factors. Whether it is a full or partial denture, the goal is to reduce or eliminate lateral forces and attempt to transmit forces parallel to the long axis of teeth. When constructing removable partial dentures, the ideal abutment teeth will be caries free, have good crown-to-root ratio, and be periodontally stable. The best teeth often will be maxillary canines and mandibular premolars. When designing your prosthesis, consider the necessary support, retention, stability, and esthetic requirements.

Review of Kennedy Classifications will help determine your success. With Kennedy Class III, you will have abutment teeth mesial and distal to the edentulous area. This will provide the best stability in most cases. With Kennedy Class II, you will have one free edentulous area, and movement will be greater, with less stability. With Kennedy Class I, you will have a bilateral edentulous area, with the least stability and the most movement along with highest degree of patient dissatisfaction. In most cases, the patient will have more difficulty functioning with a lower removable partial denture than with an upper partial denture.

When creating treatment plans for full dentures, please make sure you review with your patients the fact that they will need denture adhesive for a more secure fit. The advantage here is if they do not need it, you look good. If they do, they will not be surprised. I recommend informing patients that ideally, they would benefit from two to six implants on the upper or lower arch or both arches for the best and most secure fit. Mention that the placement of implants reduces the need for relines and in many cases reduces the bone loss caused by resorption due to disuse atrophy. This is an important concept to make sure your patients understand, adding that in time without dental implants, patients will have more and more bone loss. Their current and future dentures will fit poorly, causing many more problems and discomfort.

A word of caution regarding patients who come to you and only want a reline: once you do a reline on a patient who has had dentures for a long time, you will be irreversibly changing his or her denture, which can cause problems. I strongly recommend that you consider a new prosthesis first so you never touch his or her original denture. I find that patients who have had dentures for a long time develop a feel for them, much like an old pair of blue jeans. The dentures look bad and are beat up but still feel good, and it takes a long time for Mr. or Ms. Smith to get use to the new pair of jeans or new denture.

For the new dentist making a treatment plan for dentures, remember that the acrylic base can come in different shades, including black pigmentations. Often I see dentures in which the fit is nice, the shade and mold of the teeth are nice, but the acrylic shade does not match the patient's skin complexion. Please consider this in your treatment plan.

16. Fixed Prosthesis

Wᴛʜ ᴀʟʟ ᴅᴇɴᴛᴀʟ care and treatment, please start with complete records before beginning treatment. Complete records will include a full series of radiographs, Panorex, upper and lower impressions and bite, along with diagnostic intra- and extraoral photos. You should also evaluate your patient's range of motion and any popping, clicking, or crepitus in the right and left TMJ. Both joints should be pain-free upon palpation along with pain-free muscles of mastication. You should not start your treatment unless you have diagnostic wax-ups and a soft-shell Omnivac for provisional temporaries. You should have mounted study models and evaluate interocclusal arch space to determine whether you have enough room for the pontic or pontics. Will you be able to provide proper tooth reduction of the abutments to satisfy the needs of esthetics, retention, and resistance? You should consider double-retraction cord, starting with double zero first and then size zero second, along with full arch impressions, and I do not recommend triple trays for final impressions especially when taking an impression on multiple preparations or when a patient has a difficult or unstable occlusion, and then have a bite in centric occlusion.

Shade should be selected before preparation takes place. Discuss whether the patient will be having metal occlusion or porcelain occlusion, along with the type of material being used again prior to starting treatment. I suggest on all second and third molars you consider all-metal occlusion, and for everything else, you consider zirconium material. Whenever possible, avoid long-span bridges, avoid having a terminal abutment that has been root canaled, and make sure your patient understands what will be necessary for postinsertion maintenance. Many patients do not understand that self-threaders will be necessary to floss and maintain hygiene. When making a treatment plan, please make sure that you have a good path of insertion and that after cementation, postoperative bitewings are taken to document marginal seal. Any patient investing in a fixed prosthesis should be aware that a night guard should be considered after insertion. Every twelve to twenty-four months, postinsertion radiographs should be taken to document marginal integrity.

The fit of your prosthesis is determined by two factors. One is occlusal seat and the other is marginal seal. Remember, both are interrelated. The marginal seal is related to the film thickness of the cementing medium, which in most cases is between ten and thirty microns The goal should be to keep your marginal opening as small as possible. In most cases, eighty microns or less would be considered acceptable. Your margins will be determined by the material chosen and esthetics, along with the retention needed. In a full metal crown, you could use a feathered edge, bevel, or chamfer. In a ceramic-fused-to-metal restoration with metal collar, you could use a shoulder with a bevel or a chamfer. In a ceramic fused to metal with a ceramic margin, a shoulder type of margin will be needed. In an all-ceramic restoration, a shoulder type of margin should be done. You can elect to consider a canti-lever type of design, but you are always better off avoiding that method if possible. However, if it is necessary, never cantilever more than one tooth per fixed prosthesis, attempt to keep the size of the pontic to the size of a premolar, and eliminate any lateral forces. If possible when placing your margins, always keep the restoration margins at the free-gingival margin or above. In many cases, this situation will be unacceptable for many patients so attempt to stay away from the attachment apparatus as much as possible or at least maintain a three-millimeter distance. When this is not possible, you should discuss with your patient the need for crown lengthening.

Reviewing tooth reduction, in most cases two millimeters of reduction will keep you safe. You should have enough room in that case for all materials to provide proper esthetics and strength. Failure to provide proper reduc-tion on your preparations is, in my opinion, the single biggest problem I see in our practice day in and day out. It is so common that I suggest you inform every patient that root-canal treatment will most likely be necessary prior to starting treatment, allowing you the ability to reduce enough tooth structure without worry of pulpal irritation.

When deciding on the shade of your prosthesis, remember hue, value, and chroma. Hue refers to color of fami-lies, such as red or green. Value refers to lightness or darkness as it relates to a scale from black to white. Chroma refers to the saturation of a color. When designing your pontic, consider the following factors: the edentulous ridge; the opposing occlusal surface; musculature of the tongue, cheeks, and lips; along with form, function, and appear-ance. This will provide comfort, support, and conformity to the food-flow pattern. Several options to consider are the sanitary pontic, in which space is between the pontic and ridge. The saddle pontic covers the ridge labio-lingually. The modified ridge design uses a ridge lap for minimal ridge contact, while the labial contact is usually to the height of the ridge contour with a straight emergence profile. Finally, when designing and planning your case, pay attention to the emergence profile, which is the shape of the marginal aspect of a tooth or restoration as it re-lates to the angulation of the tooth or restoration as it emerges from the gingiva. Failure to have a proper emergence profile is a very common mistake, and in most cases, the emergence profile is overcontoured due to lack of adequate tooth reduction in your preparation.

17. ESTHETICS

IN ALL CASES, every patient is looking for his or her restoration to be esthetically pleasing or invisible to the human eye. The goals should be function and beauty. This section presents some guidelines to consider when attempting to achieve these goals. In many cases, you should be treating and assessing not just the teeth and gingival tissue that surrounds the teeth but also the lips, cheeks, and face. In general, women with large eyes, high cheekbones, full lips, and small chins will have esthetically pleasing faces.

When considering an esthetic case, which in my opinion is every case, you should consider the following.

LIP LINE, WHICH CAN CREATE A POSITIVE OR NEGATIVE APPEARANCE

This is the relationship of the upper incisors and the free-gingival margin to the upper lip at rest and while smiling. We can categorize the lip line as low, medium, or high. With a low lip line, only a small portion of the upper anterior incisors shows while smiling. With a medium upper-lip line, about one-third of the upper anterior teeth show, along with the gingival papilla. The high upper-lip line shows all of the upper anterior teeth while smiling and the gingiva.

Often, the most difficult esthetic problems will be in patients with a high lip line so be aware of this prior to treatment. A few options to consider given the high lip-line condition are orthognathic surgery, orthodontic intrusion, surgical crown lengthening, and, in some case, Botox injections.

Another important aspect to consider is the smile line. This is a series of parallel lines, providing balance to the face. It is made up of a series of horizontal lines across an individual's face: the maxillary incisal plane, gingival margin contour plane, interpupillary plane, eyebrow plane, and lip commissure plane. When examining the face, these five planes should be parallel in a well-balanced face. A worthy goal to attempt is creating a maxillary incisal line that is parallel to the line formed by the curve of the inner border of the lower lip. When examining your patient, consider the shapes of the upper central incisors. If you were to tip these teeth upside down, they would normally mimic the shape of that individual's face—square, oval, or triangular.

We should also consider dental proportions in our treatment plans by understanding that in a well-balanced smile, the ratio of width to height of a central incisor should have a width that is 80 percent of the height. This means that if the average central incisor width from mesial to distal is between eight point three millimeters and nine point three millimeters, the average length of the central incisor is between ten point four millimeters and eleven point two millimeters. On average, the lateral incisor will be one and a half to three millimeters smaller than a central incisor, and the cuspid will be one to one half millimeters wider than a lateral incisor. What we are really talking about is the divine proportion, or the golden proportion rule. This means a ratio of upper lateral to upper central is 1:1.6. You should keep in mind, though, that several studies have indicated only about 17 percent of the population falls into this golden proportion rule. Still, if possible, strive to create this balance.

You should also evaluate the contact points on the upper anterior teeth. Going from central incisors to cuspid, these interproximal contacts should gradually move gingival and parallel to the horizontal facial lines discussed above. Contact points will also help determine interdental embrasure areas, and by understanding this, you hope to avoid the dark triangles that occur when the dental papilla does not fill in the contact area. If your interdental contact point from crest of bone to contact is less than five millimeters, in most cases you can avoid the dark triangle appearance. If the distance is going to be more than five millimeters, you should be aware that often the dark triangle will be present.

The gingival contour and morphology should also be evaluated and reviewed. Keep in mind that the axial inclination, or zenith, of the free-gingival margin should be distal to the long axis of the upper incisors. When reviewing your treatment plan, please take the time to evaluate every one of the above parameters. If you do, your final result will be much better, and patient satisfaction will greatly improve. Showing knowledge in such areas will provide the confidence your patient is looking for when choosing a doctor for cosmetic care and treatment.

Cosmetic treatment planning would hardly be comprehensive if I did not address tooth whitening. Remember, all whitening works along with all techniques. The real key is to underpromise and overdeliver. I strongly recommend you inform patients that teeth with crowns, bridges, and restorations will be poor candidates for tooth whitening. I also suggest informing patients that the prediction of color change, at best, is a guess and is not permanent. Teeth with recession, in my opinion, are usually a contraindication due to sensitivity. After more than twenty years of providing tooth-whitening services, I am not a raving fan because I feel only a very small percentage of patients are ideal candidates for it. Such patients are those who do not smoke or drink colored beverages, such as cola and red wine, and have had very few restorations, preferably no anterior restorations or recessions. When that criteria has been met, then I say go for it. Make sure your patient understands that every six to twenty-four months, additional tooth whitening will need to be done. All options can potentially be successful, and you should have in-office options, tray options, light-enhanced options, or any combination thereof, informing patients that often they will experience postbleaching sensitivity, which can last anywhere from a few hours to a few weeks. Please also inform patients to drink colorless liquids for two hours after the tooth-whitening procedure.

18. MOUTH GUARDS

ALMOST EVERYONE WOULD agree that there is a huge benefit from wearing a proper-fitting and well-constructed athletic mouth guard. We can argue with the literature about whether a correctly made mouth guard can prevent concussions, but we know the debate is ongoing. However, it is certainly clear that a correctly constructed mouth guard can reduce the intensity of a concussion and can reduce the severity of injury to the teeth and peri-oral structures. Let's first review some data: around 75 percent of oral injuries occur in patients who do not wear a mouth guard. It is estimated that about 12 percent of all high school athletes will sustain some type of oral or facial injury. So let us try to reduce the severity of such injuries and educate our patients, parents, and coaches. Some sports activities that would benefit from athletes wearing an athletic mouth guard are baseball, basketball, boxing, rugby, hockey, squash, soccer, ski racing, racquetball, tennis, lacrosse, karate, judo, volleyball, football, bicycling, and skating. Mouth-guard design can be broken down into stock, boil-and-bite, vacuum custom, and heat-pressure multilaminated types.

The stock mouth guard is an over-the-counter-type mouth guard. This type offers the least protection, and it is held in place by constant biting pressure. It often dislodges on impact. It is difficult to speak while wearing it and uncomfortable. In most cases, it should not be recommended by a healthcare professional.

The boil-and-bite type is the most common type of mouth guard, and it also is purchased over the counter. After it is heated up, it is molded in the mouth to adapt to the patient's teeth and periodontal tissue. Its major disadvantage is its occlusal thickness, which is decreased between 70–99 percent during forming. It also provides a false sense of security to patients and parents. I don't feel this type of mouth guard should be recommended by healthcare professionals. I tell parents and patients that it is like wearing a seat belt incorrectly; you may feel safe, but you are not.

The vacuum and custom-built mouth guards also have the drawback of the occlusal thickness thinning by about 25 percent during construction. They tend to need replacing regularly, and they do not provide proper protection for prolonged periods. The heat-pressure multilaminated mouth guards, on the other hand, are the best by far. They are fabricated with a special high-heat, pressure-forming machine with a maximum of six atmospheres of pressure. There are several advantages with this type, such as precise adaptation, negligible deformation, the ability to thicken any area as required due to laminating capabilities, and the ability to customize each mouth guard according to the sport and level of competition. Athletes also have the ability to insert a hard polycarbonate layer between the soft ethyl vinyl acetate materials for additional protection. These guards achieve constant occlusal separation and occlusal balance. Additionally, these mouth guards do not interfere with breathing and speech, rounding out just some of their advantages.

The following are some guidelines for treatment planning a correct mouth guard. Active youth involved with contact-sport activities from mixed dentition up to age fourteen would benefit from three millimeters of soft EVA plus two millimeters of soft EVA. Active adults involved in contact sports would be best off with three millimeters of soft EVA plus three millimeters of soft EVA. This plan will work for most recreational-level adult sports.

Active professionals would be best off with three millimeters of soft EVA, two millimeters of polycarbonate, and three millimeters of soft EVA, which will work nicely for most contact sports at the professional level. Individuals participating in martial arts should consider nine millimeters of soft EVA, in situations in which intentional contact to the face will occur.

If you have to make a treatment plan for class-three occlusal-type cases, consider making the mouth guard on the lower arch. In patients with edentulous areas, consider bimaxillary or a double mouth guard for proper retention. For construction, please take full upper and lower impressions and a construction bite, which should be sent to your dental lab if made outside of your dental office. The construction bite is done with pink baseplate wax heated at 140 degrees; the wax should be folded into thirds and trimmed so that it only covers molars to cuspid, leaving the anterior teeth visible. In most cases, you will want three to five millimeters of space between the upper and lower anterior teeth. If you follow these guidelines, you will be providing a great service, reducing injuries, and creating enormous goodwill with your patients.

19. Posttreatment Records

Often this area is neglected, yet many times it can be just as important if not more important than an office's original records. Your clinical notes should be complete and detailed, and postoperative radiographs and diagnostic photos should be complete as well. I suggest you save your models in storage or have them digitized for storage, keeping the originals.

When completing dental implant cases, please document type of implant, size of implant, location of implant, and lot number. When completing a crown and bridge, document the material used in the restoration, and be sure it matches the dental insurance code used. In addition, document the cement medium used to retain your restoration, along with postinsertion bitewings and periapical if indicated. I also recommend saving your laboratory prescriptions, documenting the shade chosen.

When forced to release your dental records, please make sure you have reviewed those records before they are sent out. Make sure your radiographs are dated and labeled right and left, including which teeth are involved. Your charts should look and be professional; they are a reflection on you and your organization.

20. FOLLOW-UP CARE

I STRONGLY RECOMMEND POSTINSERTION exams within seven to fourteen days for all insertions. This includes dentures, partial dentures, and single-unit and multiunit crowns and bridges. I suggest postoperative follow up in seven to ten days for all types of dental surgery and postinsertion exams within twenty-four hours in the case of immediate dentures and/or partial dentures. Of all the follow-up care, the most important is the phone call at the end of the day to see how your patient is doing.

With root canals, I suggest following up in six months with a periapical radiograph and then again at one year, two years, and onward as needed. I recommend the following: "Mr. or Ms. Smith, I am sorry to bother you, but I just wanted to see how you are feeling. If you are having any problems, I can see you tomorrow morning." Short and sweet.

21. Raving Fan

I N THE END, your goal should be to make both your staff and your patients become raving fans. Simply stated, it is to be so good at what you are doing that your staff and your patients cannot help but tell friends and family about your practice, service and care.

REFERENCES

T HE FOLLOWING ARE sources from which many of my ideas have been derived and to whom true credit should be given.

Advanced Bone Grafting at the Medical University of South Carolina Dr. John Russo

Advanced TMJ Level I Diagnosis to Splint Construction

Clinician's Endodontic Handbook, third edition, by Thom C. Dumsha, MS, DDS, MS, and James L. Gutmann, DDS, FACD, FICD

Clinical Periodontology and Implant Dentistry, fourth edition, by Jan Lindhe

Contemporary Oral and Maxillofacial Surgery, fourth edition, by Peterson, Ellis, Hupp, and Tucker

Dental Secrets, third edition, by Stephen T. Sonis, DMD, DMSc

Evaluation, Diagnosis, and Treatment of Occlusal Problems by Dr. Peter E. Dawson

The International Association of Orthodontics seminars

Invisible Esthetic Ceramic Restorations by Sidney Kina and August Bruguera

Manual of Clinical Periodontics, second edition, by Francis F. Serio, DMD, MS, MBA, and Charles E. Hawley, DDS, PhD

Oral Surgery for the General Dentist by Lawrence I. Gaum, DDS, FADSA, FICD

The Progressive Orthodontic seminars

Space Maintainers Dental Lab

Tufts University of School of Dental Medicine, Department of Restorative Dentistry

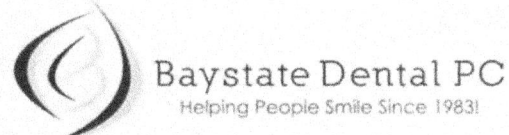

What you should know about Restorations

We can offer you four options to have a restoration completed. You can have Gold, Amalgam (Silver), Composite (tooth-colored), or Porcelain (Inlays/Onlays).

A. <u>Gold Restorations:</u> usually take two or more visits and can be costly. Many times gold fillings are noticeable in the mouth due to their yellow gold color.

B. <u>Amalgam (silver) Restorations:</u> have been around for many years and can be completed in one visit. This type of restoration is also noticeable in the mouth, and they do have a concentration of mercury in them. They are most commonly covered by insurance because they have been used for decades.

C. <u>Composite (Tooth-Colored) Restorations:</u> can be completed in one visit. They are beneficial to your mouth because they bond to the teeth, adding strength. They are very pleasing to the eye because they are tooth-colored but can stain and discolor over time.

D. <u>Porcelain (inlays/onlays) Restorations:</u> is dentistry's newest technology. They are completed in two visits. These restorations are hardly noticeable in the mouth due to the shade design to match and blend to your natural tooth color, and are bonded in place for added strength.

Upon completion of your restoration we ask that you avoid that area of your mouth for at least one hour until the anesthesia wears off and don't use dental floss for 24 hours.

As with any restoration you may experience some sensitivity. It is not unusual for symptoms to last for up to 3 months. This is typical with certain restorations. If your symptoms persist we have three options available to you. With moderate sensitivity we could place a medicated filling in the tooth for 6-8 weeks. If the tooth becomes asymptomatic then a final restoration would be placed or your tooth may require a root canal or extraction.

Insurance is not guaranteed to cover <u>any</u> of these treatments, please ask one of our friendly office members for an estimate of your out-of-pocket costs with your personal insurance plan.

Estimated fee before insurance $_____due on the day of treatment. For teeth numbers _____If payment in full cannot be made on the day of service please contact our financial coordinator before your appointment to make financial arrangements. Our computer automatically adds finance charges on unpaid balances.

Patient name (print): _____

Patient Signature: _____Date_____

Doctor Signature: _____Date_____

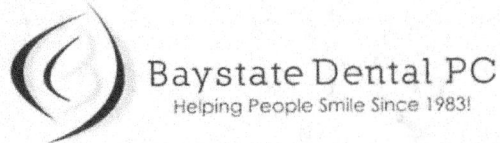

Baystate Dental is continually looking for advances to ensure that we are providing the optimal level of oral health care to our patients. We are concerned about the potential for oral cancer in every patient.

One American dies every hour from oral cancer. Late detection of oral cancer is the primary cause that both the incidence and mortality rates of oral cancer continue to increase. As with most cancers, age is the primary risk factor for oral cancer. Tobacco and alcohol use are other Major predisposing risk factors but more than 25% of oral cancer victims have no such lifestyle risk factors. Studies also suggest that human papillomavirus (HPV 16/18) plays a role in more than 20% of oral cancer cases. Oral cancer risk by patient profile is as follows:

INCREASED RISK: patients 18-39 (male and female); sexually active patients any age (HPV 16/18)

HIGH RISK: patients age 40 and older (male and female); tobacco users (ages 18-39, any type within 10 years)

HIGHEST RISK: patients age 40 and older (male and female) with lifestyle risk factors (tobacco and/or alcohol use); patients with a history of oral cancer or other cancers.

We have incorporated VELscope Vx into our oral screening standard of care. We find that using VELscope Vx along with a standard oral cancer examination improves the ability to identify suspicious areas at their earliest stages. VELscope Vx is similar to proven early detection procedures for other cancers such as mammography, Pap smear and PSA. VELscope Vx is a simple and painless examination that gives the best chance to find any oral abnormalities at the earliest possible stage. Early detection of pre-cancerous tissue can minimize or eliminate the potentially disfiguring effects of oral cancer and possibly save your life. *The VELscope Vx exam will be offered to you annually.*

This enhanced examination is recognized by the American Dental Association code revision committee as CDT-2007/08 procedure code D0431; however, this exam *might not* be covered by your insurance. The fee for this enhanced examination is $45.00. Patient Obligation $20

☐**YES**. *I authorize the clinician to perform the VELscope Vx exam along with the standard oral cancer examination. I accept financial responsibility for this enhanced examination.*

☐**NO**: *I would prefer not to have the VELscope Vx exam at this time.*

I hereby release from liability Baystate Dental, their doctors/associates, hygienists, employees or agents from any injury I may currently, or in the future, suffer as a result of my refusal to proceed with this enhanced oral cancer examination.

Print Name: _____

Signature: _____ Date: _____

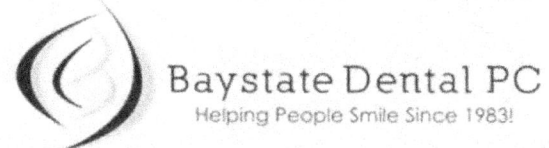

SEDATION CONSULTATION APPOINTMENT CHECKLIST

_____1. Put patient's name and date of birth into monitor

_____2. Have patient use the restroom

_____3. Seat patient and ask if patient has a business card for any and all medical doctors they may have. If they do, ask to borrow them and make a photocopy of any and all cards. If they do not have business card get the name and telephone numbers of each doctor.

_____4. Give Patient clipboard and pen with sedation consent forms to read and sign.

_____5. While patient is reading/signing consent forms, call medical doctor's office to get their exact mailing address, with zip code, telephone number and fax number. Get the name of whomever was giving the information. Write name/address/telephone numbers in space provided on next page.

_____6. After patient signs consent forms, place blood pressure cuff on **Left Arm** and pulse oximeter on **Right index finger.**

_____7. Start blood pressure and record for three(3) cycles~approximately 15 minutes.

_____8. While monitoring patient, photocopy Request for Anesthesia Request Form and After Treatment Instructions form. **KEEP ORIGINALS** and place in chart. Put copies into letterhead envelope for patient.

_____9. Have appointment card and Sedation Instructions sheet ready to fill in.

_____10. Have Prescriptions ready. (If warranted, patient needs antibiotic prescription to start the day before the appointment)

_____11. Using a tourniquet, identify vein to be used for venipuncture. Record the location of vein on venipuncture form (antecubital/hand). Or have ready for Doctor.

_____12. Review with paitent:
    1. **NOTHING** to eat or drink for 8 hours prior to IV sedation.
    2. Regular daily morning medications (blood pressure pills, etc) can be taken with a **SIP** of water.
    3. Patient **MUST** have an escort to drive them to and from the office on the day of surgery. **PATIENT CANNOT DRIVE!!**

_____13. After patient is scheduled for sedation appointment, photocopy appointment card and Sedation Instructions sheet. Place originals in letterhead envelop for patient; photocopy placed in chart.

_____14. After patient leaves, put chart with Medical Consultation form on Doctor's desk to be filled out.

_____15. Medical Consultation form is completed, photocopy form and place in chart. Take original form and fax to all medical doctors of record.

_____16. Place this sheet in patient's chart.

Medical Doctor(s) information to be recorded on next sheet.
THIS MUST BE COMPLETED!!!!

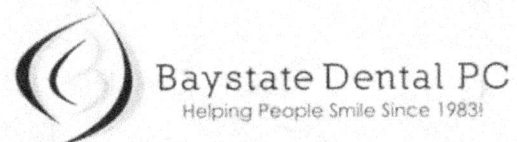

Baystate Dental PC
Helping People Smile Since 1983!

Consent for Anesthesia/Conscious/Oral Sedation

Patient Name: _____ Date: _____

Address: _____

This is my consent and authorization to administer nitrous oxide for conscious sedation, as deemed necessary, to complete the appropriate dental procedures.

I am aware that the following are possible risks and complications which may accompany this sedation and I have been informed of the nature of this sedation by one of the staff.

I understand the nature and usual effects of conscious sedation may include drowsiness, disturbances in coordination and thought processes, amnesia for recent events, and nausea.

The following are risks and complications of conscious sedation, which include but are not limited to: allergic or sensitivity reaction; aspiration; reaction or injury to the liver and kidneys; disturbance of cardiac rhythm; myocardial infraction; cardiac arrest; injury to mouth, lips, and or teeth due to the establishment or maintenance of sedation.

Nitrous oxide sedation will not be administered if you are pregnant. I affirm that I am not pregnant and release the Doctors for any liability if I find that I am.

We require that someone that is of driving age accompany the patient in case of prolonged drowsiness.

I consent to the conscious sedation and understand the complications. I also understand that I get additional explanations before or during the treatment, merely by asking.

Date: _____

Signature of Patient or Guardian: _____

Signature of Witness: _____

Signature of Doctor: _____

Start Time:					
Finish Time:					
Vitals Before	HR:		BP:		Respiration:	
Vitals After	HR:		BP:		Respiration:	
	%O2:		%N2O:			
Type and Amount of Local Anesthesia:					

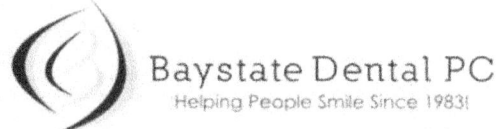

Baystate Dental PC
Helping People Smile Since 1983!

Pre-OP and Post-OP Instructions for Sedation

The following are some points of information for considering the options at Baystate Dental for patients who have mild to moderate, to even severe anxiety and dental phobic conditions.

Presently, our office has behavior modifications where we try to work with the patient over longer periods of time and slowly reduce your fear and anxiety so that dental treatment is not a major event in your life.

The next option we offer is inhalation sedation. This is where you would breathe a combination of Nitrous Oxide and Oxygen. There are almost no problems associated with this sedation. It gives you a sedation type of feeling and can reduce your anxiety significantly and seems to be most effective on those patients with mild anxiety. Contra indications would be patients who are on psychotropic drugs, have psychiatric problems, or are pregnant. In most cases, unless you have a severe upper respiratory infection or problem, this option will provide you with a level of sedation for mild to moderate treatment that needs to be done, in a very pleasing manner. The preoperative instructions are to arrive at your dental appointment about 30 minutes before your scheduled appointment time. Once the medication and treatment is completed, you would be able to get in the car and drive and you could resume your normal diet and activities. There is a fee for this service.

A deeper level of sedation is oral sedation where we use a combination of drugs in a pill form. This can also be done in combination with the Nitrous Oxide to give a slightly deeper level of sedation. The advantages of this is there are no needles involved with the administering of the medications, however, for normal routine dental care, an injection of Xylocain of Novocain type is still necessary to provide analgesic effect to have the appointment in a pain free manner. There is a fee for this service. You also must be accompanied by an adult and you should not drive for 4 to 6 hours after your treatment and you should also be monitored at home. You should also have nothing to eat or drink 4-6 hours prior to your appointment.

The next level, which is even deeper is IV sedation. In the IV sedation, we will inject a drug into your vein and that drug will put you into an even deeper level of sedation and for people who are extremely phobic, this is quite helpful. We ask you not wear fingernail or toe nail polish, please arrive 30 minutes ahead of your scheduled appointment, and that you wear loose clothing (short sleeve shirt or Jonny) so that you can be monitored appropriately. We also ask you wear no earrings, no pierced body parts, so that monitoring equipment is effective and allows us access to monitor you. We also ask that you have nothing to eat or drink for at least 4-6 hours prior to the appointment. You cannot be pregnant, not be on any psychotropic drugs that could have an adverse effect. If you are, please discuss this situation with the doctor prior to scheduling your appointment. You must have someone drive you to your appointment and home and not for 24 hours after your appointment. Please do not smoke or drink alcohol for at least 24 hours after. You also must have someone with you for at least 4 to

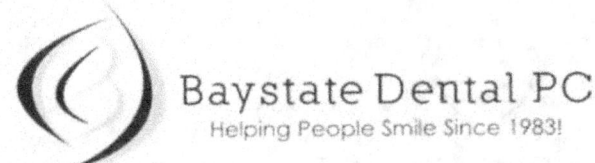

Baystate Dental PC
Helping People Smile Since 1983!

6 hours after your appointment to monitor you for any potential problems that could occur. The most common problem is dizziness and lightheaded and may require assistance walking. We also suggest your diet be light and soft after the sedation appointment for no chance of choking. There is a fee for this service. This appointment must be prepaid to be scheduled and is non-refundable. The reason for this is many of our phobic patients, find that at the last minute for a variety of reasons, they are unable to cope with their decisions and they cancel these appointments, delaying treatment for others and creating unnecessary cost for our organization.

For the deepest level of sedation is general anesthesia, which is not done in our office, but is done at the local hospitals. A tube is placed either down your throat or down your nose, providing you the ability to breath while your dental appointment is being performed in a hospital setting. Our fee to schedule you in the hospital is $495 and then there are the other fees for the dental treatment and other fees associated with the hospitalization for a Day Stay patient. In almost all cases, you would go home that same day, but if we feel you would be better monitored by keeping you over night, then we will discharge you when appropriate.

Almost 98% of all dental cases associated with fear and anxiety can be treated with inhalation, oral, or IV sedation and the most severe cases, require general anesthesia. If you need additional information, we would be happy to provide you with that during your consultation visits, if necessary. We hope the following has provided you with insight to make your procedure go as smooth as possible.

Most people who choose these sedation methods for complicated issues, such as dental extractions and implant surgery, but many times will also elect this for hygiene appointments and simple restorations, based on their level of anxiety and fear.

Baystate Dental has explained all risks, benefits, costs and options and we have given you, the patient, the opportunity to ask any questions.

Date: _____

Signature of Patient or Guardian: _____

Signature of Witness: _____

Signature of Doctor: _____

JUST ENOUGH TO BE GREAT IN YOUR DENTAL PROFESSION

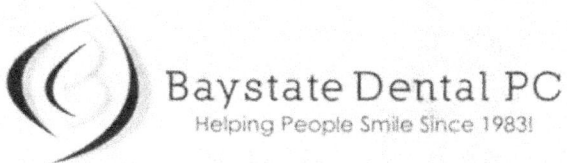

Baystate Dental PC
Helping People Smile Since 1983!

Instructions to Patients Scheduled for Conscious Sedation

1. Nothing by mouth for eight (8) hours prior to the planned procedure, except for medications with a sip of water, if so advised by your doctor.

2. You must be accompanied by a competent adult who is able to drive and can escort you home. This adult must arrive with you, wait in the waiting area during the procedure and leave with you when you are discharged.

3. Any change in your medical status must be reported to the doctor on the day of the planned procedure. These may include cold or flu, positive pregnancy test or suspected pregnancy, newly discovered allergy, newly diagnosed medical condition or the addition of new medication or cessation of medication previously prescribed.

4. We ask that you wear loose fitting clothing so that we are able to apply our blood pressure cuff and monitors. Sometimes tight fitting clothing including jeans can restrict your breathing. No contact lens, make up, nail polish or body piercings should be worn for this appointment.

You will need at least 30 minutes after the procedure to recover from the effects of sedation. Discharge will be delayed if you doctor does not fee you are ready to leave his/her care. In the rare event that you are unable to fill the requirements of a safe discharge, admission to the hospital may be necessary. If you have any questions prior to the procedure, please do not hesitate to call.

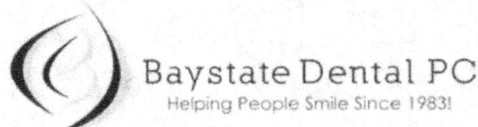

Baystate Dental PC
Helping People Smile Since 1983!

Informed Consent for IV Sedation

Dr./Drs._____ has reviewed the risks, benefits, and alternatives of IV Sedation. After being informed of the risks, benefits, and alternatives, you have agreed to allow staff and doctors to perform the following procedures: _____.

IV Sedation will allow the doctors to provide a drug intravenously that will place you in a state of relaxation that will take the high anxiety and high fear patient and hopefully make their dental experience more acceptable. As with any medical procedure, there are risks which could be death and permanent disability. Although those are extremely rare those risks are possible and you have been thoroughly made aware of what those risks are along with any additional options.

Because your state of consciousness may be somewhat altered, and treatment plans may need change, it is imperative that you have given Baystate Dental's doctors and staff permission to modify and change discussed treatment plans as they feel is most appropriate and best for your care. In most cases, we will attempt to adhere to out treatment plan as strictly as possible so that there are no surprises or changes.

You have been informed that there is a fee for this sedation treatment and the monitoring and that fee is based on the first hour and then in increments of 15 minutes. In preparation for your treatment, it is imperative that you have nothing to eat or drink for four hours prior to your IV sedation procedure. You must wear loose clothing so that the doctors and staff will have access for monitoring equipment. It is imperative that any changes in your medical history and any medications that you are on are brought to the staff's attention prior to treatment.

It is requested that you arrive to your appointment 10-15 minutes prior to your scheduled time in preparation for your care and treatment. It is mandatory that you don not show up to the appointment by yourself. You must have an adult present with you. Please use the restroom before being seated for this appointment. Our recommendation is that the adult should stay with you for the next 2-4 hours until the medication has significantly worn off.

You should not make critical decisions, work with machinery or equipment, or drive for 4-6 hours after your procedure. Sometimes artificial fingernails, heavy make-up, and jewelry can interfere with monitoring equipment and we have asked that no jewelry, no make-up, and no artificial nails be worn for the appointment. In certain instances, it is difficult to monitor your cardiovascular system, which is typically done on the wrist. In those rare cases, you may have leads or cardiovascular leads placed on your chest region. Since most patients are not familiar with these types of treatment in a dental office, please be aware that if monitoring equipment needs to be altered, you may have leads or patches placed below your right clavicle, below your left clavicle, and on the left lateral aspect or side below the breast or nipple area. We will try our best to inform you if that is necessary, however in most cases these leads will be placed on your finger and wrist to avoid any potential issues or problems.

We are pleased that you have chosen our office for your sedation techniques and will do everything in our power to make the situation as comfortable and as stress free as possible. By signing below, you understand the risks, benefits, and alternatives. Please sign and date.

Patient's signature: _____ Date: _____

Doctor's signature: _____ Date: _____

Witness's signature: _____ Date: _____

— 88 —

Conscious Sedation Pre-Procedure Record
Baystate Dental PC
1795 Main Street – Suite 215
Springfield, MA 01103
413-733-6651

Date _____ Unit _____
Patient Name_____ Doctor_____
Procedure_____ Operator_____
Diagnosis_____ Assistant_____
Time in_____ Referring/Ordering_____

ASSESSMENT

Age	Wt.	kg	□ Dentures	□ Partial Plate
Sex M F	FlO$_2$ / O$_2$	% / lpm	NPO since	

MENTAL STATUS	INTRAVENOUS		VITAL SIGNS		ALDRETE SCORE
□ Alert □ Oriented □ Disoriented	Insertion		Heart Rate	/min	Activity
□ Relaxed □ Anxious □ Agitated	Cannula	g	Rhythm		Respiration
□ Sedative / Analgesic use in the past 8 hrs	Site		Blood Pressure		Circulation
(specify):	Solution		Respirations	/min	Consciousness
□ Ethanol / Illicit Drug use in the past 8 hrs	Rate	cc/hr	SaO$_2$	%	Oxygenation
(specify):	Patency		Temperature		Total

MEDICATIONS

Current Medications:
Allergies and Adverse Reactions:

PRE-SEDATION CHECKLIST

□ ASA Physical status cleared by MD   □ History and Physical completed by MD
□ Informed Consent obtained   □ Laboratory Tests obtained
□ IV Conscious Sedation Discharge Instructions given   □ ECG completed

COMPLETED BY

Signature	Initial	Signature	Initial	Signature	Initial

PHYSICIAN

Anesthesia	
Airway	□ WNL
Respiratory	□ WNL
Cardiovascular	□ WNL
Substance Use	□ ETOH

ASA Class	I	II	III	IV	V
NPO Status	□ 6 hours food	□ 4 hours clear liquids	□ meds with sips of clear liquids	□ no restriction	
Planned Medication(s)	□ fentanyl	□ meperidine	□ midazolem	□ morphine	□ other

I have discussed the indication, benefits, risks, and alternatives to IV conscious sedation with the patient and/or responsible party and have obtained consent for conscious sedation.

Signature of examining physician: Date :   Time:

Conscious Sedation Post-Procedure Record
Baystate Dental PC
1795 Main Street – Suite 215
Springfield, MA 01103
413-733-6651

PARENTERAL						TIME							TOTAL	POST-PROCEDURE NOTES
IV (cc/hr)														

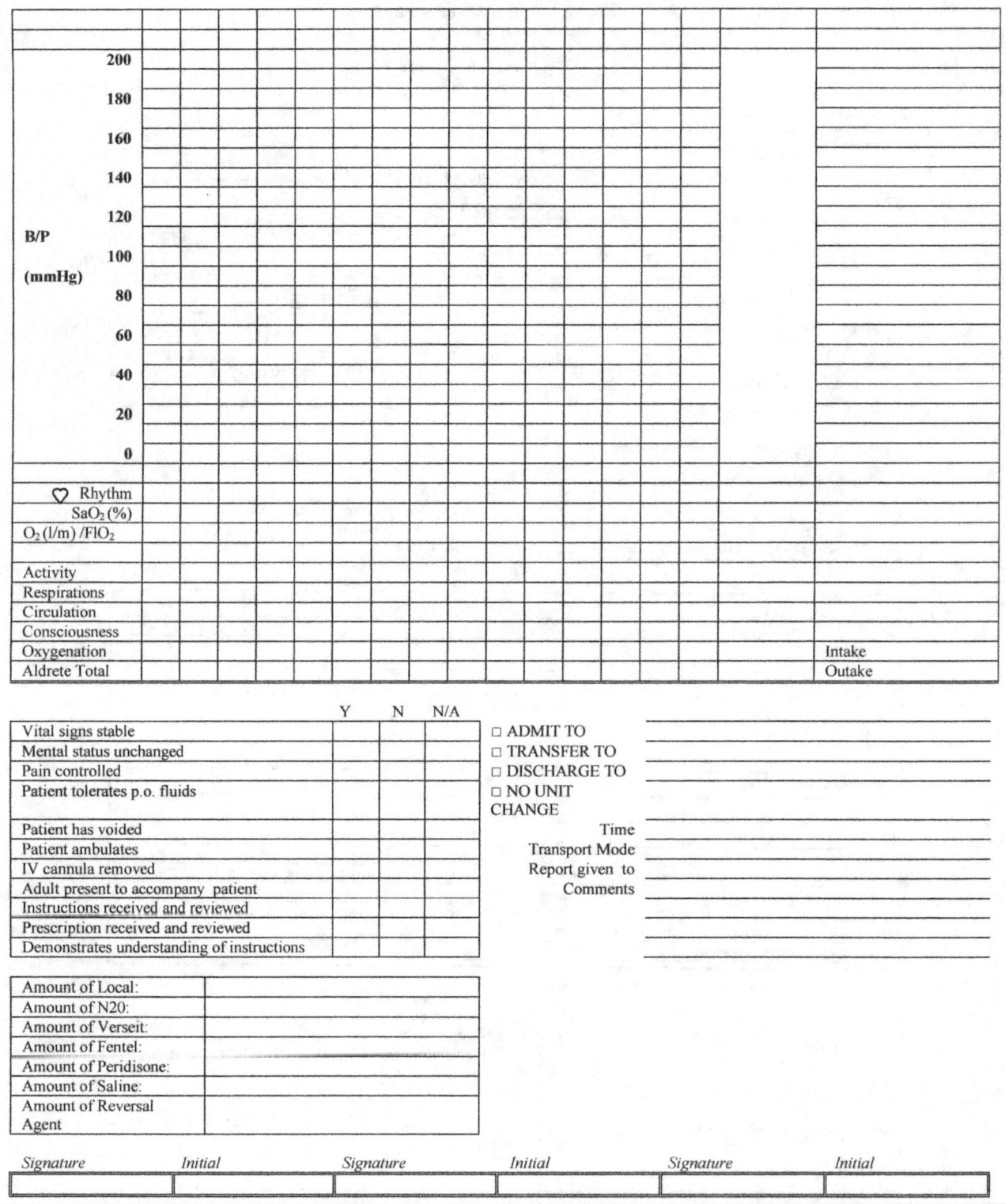

B/P (mmHg)

200
180
160
140
120
100
80
60
40
20
0

♡ Rhythm
SaO₂ (%)
O₂ (l/m) /FlO₂

Activity
Respirations
Circulation
Consciousness
Oxygenation — Intake
Aldrete Total — Outake

	Y	N	N/A
Vital signs stable			
Mental status unchanged			
Pain controlled			
Patient tolerates p.o. fluids			
Patient has voided			
Patient ambulates			
IV cannula removed			
Adult present to accompany patient			
Instructions received and reviewed			
Prescription received and reviewed			
Demonstrates understanding of instructions			

☐ ADMIT TO
☐ TRANSFER TO
☐ DISCHARGE TO
☐ NO UNIT CHANGE
Time
Transport Mode
Report given to
Comments

Amount of Local:	
Amount of N20:	
Amount of Verseit:	
Amount of Fentel:	
Amount of Peridisone:	
Amount of Saline:	
Amount of Reversal Agent	

Signature   Initial   Signature   Initial   Signature   Initial

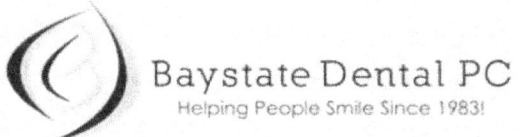

Baystate Dental PC
Helping People Smile Since 1983!

Consent for Periodontal Surgery

Patient Name: _____ Date: _____

Address: _____

This is my consent to the periodontal surgery indicated by examination and any other oral surgery deemed necessary or advisable to the planned operation. I, also agree to the use for local anesthetic and am aware of the following possible complications of surgery,

which include, but is not limited to: loss of teeth that are periodontally involved; problems with the anesthesia, drugs, and medication; the hazards of surgery include pain, bleeding, swelling, infection, possible permanent numbness or tingling of the lips, face, gum or tongue and the possibility of loss of adjacent teeth, sensitivity to remaining teeth to temperature changes, teeth may appear longer and or larger due to the surgical procedure. I also allow for the augmentation of artificial, cadaver, or animal bone and tissue substances when and if it is advisable.

I also understand that I am responsible for adequate oral hygiene and continuing visits for hygiene appointments and home care instructions, in which appropriate additional fees will be applied. I am further advised that I can get additional explanations of risks before or during the progress of any treatment simply by asking.

If you have been treated with IV and or oral Bisphosphonate drugs you should know that there is a risk of future severe complications that might happen with dental treatment. There is a small but real risk. Jawbones usually heal themselves very well and maintain their normal health. In some patients, Bisphosphonate drugs seem to affect the ability of jawbones to break down or remodel themselves. This interferes with the jaw's ability to heal itself. This risk is increased after surgery, especially from extractions, gum surgery; implant placement or other "invasive" procedures that might cause mild trauma to bone. Necrosis (dying cells) or Osteonecrosis (dying bone cells) may result and an infection may occur in the soft tissue and or inside the bone. This is a long-term process that destroys the jawbone that is often very hard or even impossible to get rid of. In some periodontal surgery cases additional surgery is necessary to be preformed. I understand that additional charges could occur.

Date: _____

Signature of Patient of Guardian: _____

Signature of Witness: _____

Signature of Doctor: _____

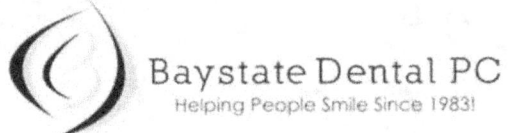

Baystate Dental PC
Helping People Smile Since 1983!

Consent for Extraction(s)

Patient Name: _____ Date: _____

Address: _____ BP _____ P_____

I authorize Dr. _____ and his/her dental team to extract teeth #_____ and to place bone grafting material. If any unforeseen condition arises in the course of the procedure calling for, in the doctor's judgment, procedures in addition to or different from those now contemplated, I further request and authorize my doctor to do whatever he/she deems advisable.

This is my consent to the treatment indicated by examination and any other oral surgery deemed necessary or advisable to the planned operation. I also agree to the use of a local anesthetic and am aware of the following possible complications of surgery, which include, but is not limited to: loss of teeth that are periodontally involved, problems with the anesthesia, drugs, and medications, the hazards of surgery include pain, bleeding, swelling, infection, possible permanent numbness or tingling of the lips, face, gums or tongue and the possibility of loss of adjacent teeth, sensitivity of remaining teeth to temperature changes, teeth may appear longer and/or larger due to the surgical procedure. In the extraction of third molars there is a minimal possibility of fracture of the lower jaw or complications with the maxillary sinus. I also allow for the augmentation of artificial, animal or human bone substances when and if it is advisable. I also understand that I am responsible for adequate oral hygiene and continuing visits for hygiene appointments and home care instructions, in which appropriate additional fees will be applied. I am further advised that I can get additional explanations of risks before or during the progress of any treatment simply by asking.

I understand that if nothing is done any of the following could occur: bone disease, lose of bone, gum tissue inflammation, infection, sensitivity, looseness of teeth followed by necessity of extraction. Also possible are temporomandibular joint (jaw) problems, headaches, referred pain to back of neck and facial muscles, and tired muscles when chewing. In addition, I am aware that if nothing is done an inability to place implants at a later date due to changes in oral or medical conditions could exist.

I understand that excessive smoking, alcohol, or blood sugar may effect gum healing. I agree to follow my doctor's home care instructions. I agree to report to my doctor for regular examinations as instructed.

My doctor has fully explained the following to me: a) the nature of my condition b) the nature and purpose of the procedure that I am now authorizing c) the nature and probability of the risks involved in the procedure, including possible complications and side effects that may result d) the benefits to be reasonably expected from the procedure e) the likely result of no treatment f) the available alternatives, including their risks and benefits. My doctor has also explained that, in addition to the specific risks involved in this procedure, there are other possible risks that accompany any surgical or diagnostic procedure. I acknowledge that my doctor has made no guarantees or assurances to me as to the result of the procedure that I am now authorizing.

My doctor has explained that there is no method to predict accurately the gum and bone healing capabilities in each patient.

To my knowledge, I have given an accurate report of my physical and mental history. I have also reported any prior allergic or unusual reactions to drugs, food, insect bites, anesthetics, pollens, dust, blood or body diseases, gum or skin reactions, abnormal bleeding or any other conditions related to my health.

If you have been treated with IV and or oral Bisphosphonate drugs to increase bone density, you should know that there is a risk of future severe complications that might happen with dental treatment. There is a small but real risk. Jawbones usually heal themselves very well and maintain their normal health. In some patients, Bisphosphonate drugs seem to affect the ability of jawbones to break down or remodel themselves. This interferes with the jaw's ability to heal itself. This risk is increased after surgery, especially from extractions, gum surgery; implant placement or other "invasive" procedures that might cause mild trauma to bone. Necrosis (dying cells) or Osteonecrosis (dying bone cells) may result and an infection may occur in the soft tissue and or inside the bone. This is a long-term process that destroys the jawbone that is often very hard or even impossible to get rid of.

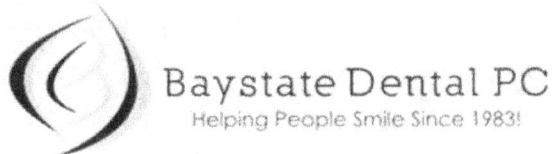

I consent to photography, filming, recording, x-rays, and additional professional staff observing the procedure to be performed for the advancement of dentistry, provided my identity is not revealed.

I certify that I have read and fully understand this authorization for treatment, that the explanations referred to in this form were made, and that all blocks or statements requiring completion were filled in before I signed my name. I further understand that the doctor has relied upon this certification in allowing this treatment to be preformed. I acknowledge that my questions about this procedure have been answered.

Date: _____

Signature of Patient of Guardian: _____

Signature of Witness:_____

Signature of Doctor: _____

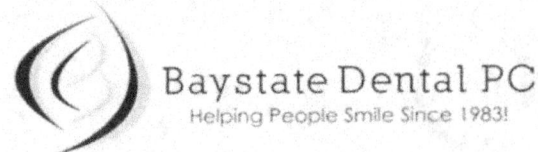

Baystate Dental PC
Helping People Smile Since 1983!

Consent for Implant Surgery and Anesthesia

PATIENT NAME: _____   DATE: _____
ADDRESS: _____

The implant surgery procedures have been explained to me and I understand what is necessary to accomplish the placement of the implant under the gums or in the bone. The Doctor has carefully examined me. To my knowledge I have given an accurate report of my health history. Any prior allergic or unusual reactions to drugs, food, insect bites, anesthetics, pollen, dust, or abnormal bleeding conditions related to my health are included.

I was informed of other methods, which would replace the missing teeth. I have tried or considered these methods and I prefer an implant to help secure the replaced missing teeth. I understand that any of the following could occur: bone disease, loss of bone, gum tissue inflammation, infections, and sensitivity, looseness of teeth followed by necessity of extraction. Also possible are temporal mandibular joint problems, headaches, and referred pain to back of neck and facial muscles, and tired muscles when chewing. I also understand that if conventional removable dentures are used, I may suffer injury to and or loss of teeth and bone as well.

The Doctor has explained that there is no method to accurately predict the gum and bone healing capabilities in each patient following the placement of the implant. I understand that smoking, alcohol, or departure from acceptable dieting practices may affect gum healing and may limit success of the implant. I agree to follow home care and diet recommendations per instructions. I agree to report to the Doctor's office for check-ups as instructed and I understand that a reasonable fee will be made for these examinations. If for any reason the Doctor deems that the implant is not serving properly it is agreed that the implant will be removed. It will be replaced by conventional prosthesis or another implant depending on the decision of the Doctor.

I have been informed and understand that occasionally there are complications of the surgery, drugs, and/or anesthesia. Pain, swelling, infection, discoloration or numbness of the lip, tongue, chin, cheek, or teeth may occur, the exact duration of which may not be determinable. The numbness may be irreversible. Also possible are inflammation of vein, injury to teeth if present, bone fracture, nasal or sinus penetration, delayed healing, and allergic reactions. It has been explained that in some patients implants fail and must be removed.

With full understanding, I authorize the Doctor to perform dental services for me, including implants and other surgery. I agree to the type of anesthesia chosen by the Doctor. I agree not to operate a motor vehicle or other hazardous device for 24 hours or until fully recovered from the effects of the anesthesia or drugs given for my care, which ever is longer.

I authorize photos, slides, x-rays, or any other viewing of my case and treatment during its progress to be used for the advancement of dentistry. I approve any modifications in design, materials, or care if in the professional judgment of the Doctor it is in my best interest. I understand that there is no warranty or guarantee to my results. I am further advised that I can get additional explanations of the risks before or during the progress of any treatment merely by asking. If additional implant surgery is necessary additional fees will be charged. I understand implants can fail, and that like natural teeth the implant must be cleaned and maintained to provide the best outcome.

DATE: _____

Signature of Patient of Guardian: _____

Signature of Doctor: _____

Signature of Witness: _____

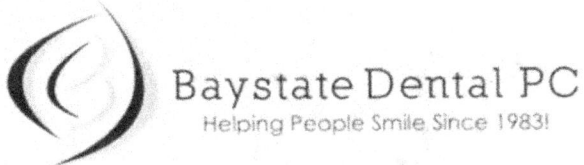

Baystate Dental PC
Helping People Smile Since 1983!

understand that my personal daily care (recommended by my doctor) and taking all prescribed medications are important to the ultimate success of the frenectomy.

The alternatives to the recommended treatment have been discussed and I understand that if no treatment will be done the possibility of advancement of my condition may result to premature loss of teeth and or impairment of my general health.

I hereby acknowledge no guarantee, warranty or assurance has been given to me that the proposed treatment should provide benefit in reducing the cause of my condition and should produce healing which will help me keep my teeth. Due to individual patient differences, however, the doctor cannot predict certainty of success. There is a risk of failure, relapse, additional treatment or worsening of my present condition, including the possible loss of certain teeth, despite the best care.

I certify that I have read and fully understand this document.

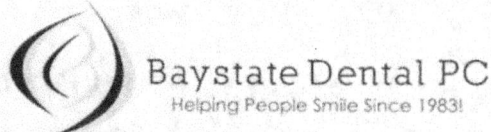
Baystate Dental PC
Helping People Smile Since 1983!

Post-Operative Instructions for Dental Surgery

The following is a list of post-operative instructions to help the healing process. Please follow these instructions after dental surgery appointments.

The main concern with any dental surgery is bleeding and pain. The following will help with both of these concerns.

1. During the first 24 hrs. after your appointment, it's important for a blood clot to form in the extraction site to stop bleeding, reduce pain and speed healing. To help the clot form, bite on the gauze pad firmly for 45 to 60 minutes after extraction. Also a dampened teabag can be used in place of the gauze due to the tannic acid in the teabag.

2. To protect the clot and avoid a painful condition called Dry Socket, don't do anything to dislodge or dissolve the clot for the first 24 hours. This means don't spit, don't suck through a straw or suck candies.
   For the first 24 hours, don't drink hot or carbonated drinks and eat hot spicy food. Avoid eating foods such as peanuts and popcorn, which may lodge in the extraction site and cause discomfort. As soon as you feel comfortable you may begin to eat normally.
   Do not smoke or drink alcohol for at least 72 hours as these drugs retard the healing process and cause post-operative complications. You may rinse gently with warm saline water (1 teaspoon of salt per glass of water) after 24 hours.

3. Limit yourself to calm activities for the first 24 hours. This protects the clot by keeping your blood pressure lower and reduce bleeding.

4. It's normal to experience some pain and discomfort for several days following an extraction. To keep swelling to a minimum, use an icebag or pack, 20 minutes on and 20 minutes off. After 24 hours you can apply moist heat to reduce swelling and soreness.

5. Unless told to do so by the physician, refrain from using aspirin compounds. Aspirin tends to prolong the bleeding time and can aggravate the healing process. To control discomfort you may use Tylenol or Tylenol type medications. Take the medication before the anesthetic wears off. If antibiotics are prescribed, continue to take them for the length of time indicated, even if the signs and symptoms of infection are gone.

6. Resume regular brushing and flossing after 24 hours, but gently clean the area around the extraction site for about a week.

7. Call our office if you have heavy or increased bleeding, you have pain or swelling that continues beyond 3 days, you develop a bad taste or odor in your mouth or a reaction to the medication prescribed.

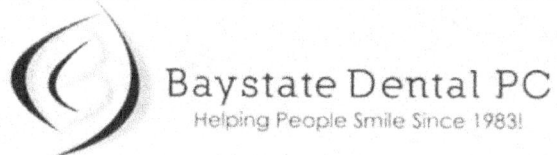

Baystate Dental PC
Helping People Smile Since 1983!

AFTER TREATMENT INSTRUCTIONS

Initial below:

_____1.   Patient **cannot** drive for 24 hour after treatment

_____2.   Patient **cannot** operate any hazardous devices for 24 hours

_____3.   A responsible person should be with the patient until he/she has fully recovered from the effects of the medications.

_____4.   Patient should **not** go up and down stairs unattended. Let the patient stay on the ground floor until recovered.

_____5.   Patient can eat whenever and whatever he/she wants.

_____6.   Patient **must drink plenty of fluids** as soon as possible.

_____7.   Patient may sleep for a long time or may be alert when he/she leaves. Attend to both alert and sleepy patient in the same manner—**DO NOT** trust him/her alone.

_____8.   **Always** hold patient's arm when walking

_____9.   Call us if you have any questions or difficulties. If you feel that your symptoms warrant a physician and you are unable to reach us, go to the closest emergency room immediately.

Following most surgical procedures, there may or may not be pain, depending on your threshold for pain. You will be provided with medication for discomfort that is appropriate for you. In most cases, a non-narcotic pain regimen will be given consisting of acetaminophen (Tylenol) and ibuprofen (Advil). These two medications <u>taken together</u> will be as effective as a narcotic without any side effects associated with a narcotic. If a narcotic has been prescribed, follow the instructions carefully. If you have any questions about these medications interacting with other medications you are presently taking, <u>please call our office first, you physician and/or your pharmacist.</u>

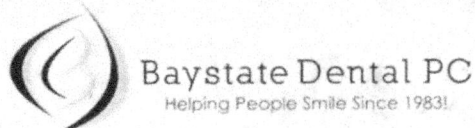

Baystate Dental PC
Helping People Smile Since 1983!

Consent for Fixed Prostheses

Patient Name: _____ Date: _____

Address: _____

The following informed consent is to provide you, the patient, with as much information as possible to protect your investment long and short term.

You have agreed to have a fixed prosthetic procedure done in your mouth. This means irreversible reduction of natural tooth structure and existing fillings. Typically this procedure is completed in two to four visits. The success of this procedure depends on the doctor's skill, techniques and the patient's ability to maintain their mouth. Excellent hygiene is extremely important to protect your investment.

Teeth that have been crowned or capped can still get periodontal (gum) disease and cavities. Either of these procedures can have a deleterious effect on the long and short-term success of your crowns or caps. To protect your investment there are a variety of techniques available to improve long-term success. Using fluoride on a daily basis, excellent hygiene (brushing and flossing properly twice daily), hygiene exams in the dental office every six months, and dental techniques such as crown root lengthening and periodontal surgery can often improve the long-term success of care. With most treatments, we hope common sense will guide you, the patient, and our staff to provide the best treatment in the most sensible fashion.

If you have questions about crown root lengthening or periodontal surgery to improve the long-term success of your fixed prosthesis, please bring this to out attention immediately. Out ultimate goal is to provide you with the best care and success.

It is imperative that you understand that periodontal surgery, root canals and fillings done after the crown and bridges have been completed may necessitate treatment to be redone, which causes the patient unnecessary expense and time. We use our expertise and common sense to try to avoid these procedures to reduce patient cost and discomfort. However, when we do this we must depend on your commitment to excellent hygiene and strongly urge you to consider having your teeth routinely cleaned, polished, examined and fluoridated every three months. Deviation from this strict course changes the outcome and increases the possibility of a remake or redo, at the patient's expense.

I hope the above has explained some of the pros and cons of your treatment. You must be aware that during fixed prosthetic procedures, as the teeth are reduced, we come close to the nerve inside the tooth. As this distance decreases, the probability of hot and cold sensitivity increases. One way to avoid this sensitivity is to root canal the tooth and remove the nerve prior to insertion of the crown. This technique can be done, however, it also increases the cost and treatment time. Our office policy is to try to maintain the teeth as vital as possible.

Should you not want any sensitivity after insertion of the crowns or bridges, root canals may be a necessary form of treatment. Another reason for considering root canal therapy prior to crowning and capping is inadequate tooth structure available for the crown to be cemented on. If this is the case, once the root canal is completed, posts, buildups and pins are used to provide adequate crown material so the crown can be cemented with adequate retention for long-term success.

Should we deviate from these procedures, which we do daily to avoid root canal therapy and additional expenses, there is a higher likelihood that the crowns may have to be re-cemented and the seal on the cement may be less than adequate.

If you have any questions or comments, please do not hesitate to call or talk with us prior to the start of treatment. We ask you not to eat anything sticky or chewy for 24 hours after the insertion of your fixed prosthesis. We then expect you to resume normal activities and maintain these teeth as you would your natural teeth

Date: _____

Signature of Patient of Guardian: _____

Signature of Witness: _____

Signature of Doctor: _____

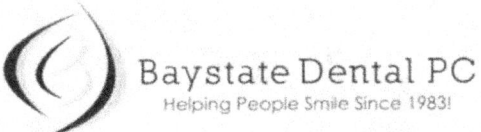

Baystate Dental PC
Helping People Smile Since 1983!

Consent for Root Canal Therapy

Patient Name: _____ Date: _____

Address: _____

1. Root canal therapy is about 95% successful. Many factors influence the treat outcome: the patient's general health, bone support around the tooth, strength of the tooth including possible fracture lines, shape and condition of the root and nerve canal (s), etc.

2. Teeth treated with root canals must be protected during treatment. We will slightly reduce the height of molar and premolar teeth during treatment to help reduce the biting force placed on these teeth. Caution should be used chewing on treated teeth since all teeth of the potential to fracture until a crown is placed.

3. The tooth may normally be sensitive following the appointments and even remain tender for a time after treatment is complete. If sensitivity persists, and does not seem to be getting better, even several weeks after the root canal is finished, please let the doctor know.

4. Fractures are one of the main reasons why root canals fail. Unfortunately, some cracks that extend from the crown down to the root are invisible and hard to detect. They can occur on uncrowned teeth from traumatic injury, biting on hard objects, habitual clenching or even just normal wear. Whether the fracture occurs before or after the root canal, it may require extraction of the tooth.

5. Since teeth with root canals are more brittle than other teeth, the dentist will probably recommend a crown to prevent future damage. This is especially important with molar and bicuspid teeth.

6. Teeth treated with root canals can still decay, but since the nerve is gone, there will be no pain. As with other teeth, the proper care of these teeth consists of good home care and periodic dental checkups.

7. With some teeth, conventional root canal therapy alone may not be sufficient. For example, if the canal(s) are severely bent or calcified, if there is substantial or long-standing infection in the bone around the roots, or if a metal file becomes separated within a canal, the tooth may remain sensitive and a surgical procedure or extraction may be necessary to resolve the problem.

8. There are alternatives to root canal therapy. They include no treatment at all (which may place you at risk), extraction with nothing to fill the space and extraction followed by a bridge, implant, or partial denture to fill the space.

9. After root canal therapy has been completed there will be a temporary filling in the tooth. You should return for final restorative or prosthetic treatment as soon as possible.

10. The nature of root canal therapy has been explained to me and I have had a chance to have my questions answered. I understand that dentistry is not an exact science and success with root canal treatment cannot be guaranteed. I understand that there are potential risks (such as swelling, sensitivity, numbness etc.) and are not limited to those discussed. Additional unknown or unspecified problems, the explanation for and the responsibility of cannot be given or assumed. In the light of the above information, I authorize the doctor to proceed with root canal treatment.

Date: _____

Signature of Patient of Guardian: _____

Signature of Witness: _____

Signature of Doctor: _____

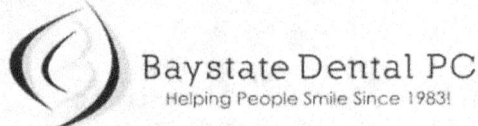

Baystate Dental PC
Helping People Smile Since 1983!

Consent for the Processing of a Partial or Denture

I, _____, give permission to Dr. _____ to process my partial or denture and go to a finish. I have been given the opportunity to wear and see my partial or denture with the teeth set in wax. I am pleased with the esthetics of the partial or denture, including, but not limited to the shape, form, positioning, and color (shade _____) of the teeth and of the framework.

I am aware that once processed, the partial or denture is finished and the teeth might have to be cut off in order to be changed in any way. This may lead to the destruction of the partial or denture and to more appointments in order to correct the problem. Therefore, if I decide later that I do not like the esthetics (look) of the teeth or of the framework, there may be a charge up to the full fee of the original partial or denture to correct the problem.

Date: _____

Signature of Patient or Guardian: _____

Signature of Witness: _____

Signature of Doctor: _____

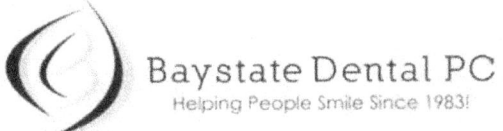

Baystate Dental PC
Helping People Smile Since 1983!

Consent for Orthodontic Treatment

Patient Name: _____ Date: _____

Address: _____

As a rule, excellent orthodontic results can be achieved with informed and cooperative patients. Thus the following information is routinely supplied to anyone considering orthodontic treatment in our office. While recognizing the benefits of a pleasing smile and healthy, functional teeth, you should also be aware that orthodontic treatment like any treatment of the body has some hazards, inconveniences, and limitations. These drawbacks seldom out weight the long-range benefits, but should be considered in making the decision to wear orthodontic appliances.

While we do not limit our practice to orthodontics only perfection is our goal. The doctor will use his knowledge, training, skill, and experience to achieve function that is esthetically pleasing, but much depends on the patient's growth patterns, genetics, oral health and cooperation.

Throughout life, tooth positions are constantly changing. This is true with all individuals regardless of whether they have worn braces or not. After orthodontic treatment, patients are subject to the same subtle changes that occur in non-orthodontic patients. In the late teens or early twenties orthodontic patients may notice slight irregularities developing in their front teeth. This is particularly true if their teeth were extremely crowded or protrusive prior to treatment. Prolonged wearing of a retainer may be the only way to prevent this if it becomes undesirable.

Decalcification (permanent markings on the teeth), tooth decay, or gum disease can occur if patients do not brush and floss their teeth properly and thoroughly. Excellent oral hygiene and daily plaque removal are musts. Sugars and between meal snacks should be eliminated. Regular check-ups with the dentist are necessary to check for decay and clean teeth. Occasionally periodontal (gum) problems present before orthodontic treatment may be worsened by the wearing of braces and require treatment.

Cold sores, canker sores, and irritation or injury to the mouth are possible while wearing braces. Allergic reactions to dental materials or medications are rare, but do occur occasionally. There may be a need for extractions of teeth, fillings, crowns, bridges, gum treatment, or other dental procedures before, during, or after orthodontic treatment.

On rare occasions the nerve of a tooth may become abscessed. A tooth that has been irritated by a deep filling or even a minor blow may require treatment.

In some instances the root ends of the teeth are shortened during treatment. This is called root resorption. Under healthy circumstances the shortened roots are no disadvantage. There is no way to foresee whether this will happen and nothing can be done to prevent this from occurring.

There is also very small chance that pain may occur in the lower jaw joints. Tooth alignment or bite corrections can usually improve tooth-related causes of jaw discomfort, but additional treatment may be required outside the realm of orthodontics.

Occasionally a person who has grown normally and in average proportion may not continue to do so. If growth becomes disproportionate, the jaw position can be affected and the original treatment objectives may have been compromised. Skeletal growth and disharmony is a biological process beyond the dentist's control.

Orthodontic treatment can succeed only through the joint cooperation of all parties involved. Together we can achieve the best possible results. In may instances, lack of cooperation in the requested use of headgear, elastics, functional orthopedic appliances, and retainers will make a successful completion of treatment impossible, or lengthen the duration of treatment.

We appreciate your confidence in selecting our office. We want you to be fully informed, so ask questions anytime. During the period of orthodontic treatment we will make models, x-rays, and photographs which may be used for professional reference and display, orthodontic journals, books, and meetings and patient education.

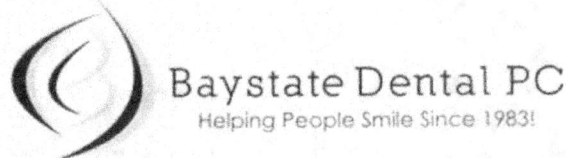

If treatment has not been completed do to relocation or change of dental office the fee will be prorated based on 24 months of 4 equal payments or % of treatment completed.

I have read and understand this letter and with this knowledge consent to treatment.

Date: _____

Signature of Patient or Guardian: _____

Signature of Witness: _____

Signature of Doctor: _____

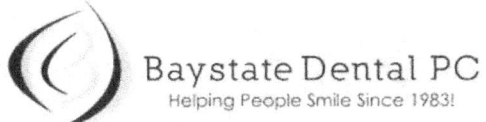

TMJ Treatment Sheet

Name: _____ Date: _____

Date of Birth: _____ Sex: M F Race: White Black Hispanic Asian Other: _____

Occupation: _____ Chief Complaint: _____

Duration of Problems: _____

When is the problem most severe? Morning Afternoon Evening Sleeping Eating No Pattern

List present medications and dose: _____

_____

1. Are you currently seeking a lawyers help for your problem?	Yes	No
2. Are you now or in the past trying to collect disability for head, neck, back, or jaw problems?	Yes	No
3. Do you have frequent headaches?	Yes	No

    a. If so, where? _____

    b. How long do they last? _____

4. Please list any trauma to any part of your body no matter how minor it may seem or how long ago it may have occurred, starting with the most recent: _____

_____

_____

5. Are your jaws clenched when you awaken from sleep?	Yes	No
6. Do you grind your teeth when you sleep?	Yes	No
7. Do you grind your teeth when you are awake?	Yes	No
8. Have you had your lower wisdom teeth removed?	Yes	No
9. Have you ever had orthodontic treatment?	Yes	No
10. Were teeth removed for orthodontic treatment?	Yes	No
11. Have you ever been treated for a bad bite?	Yes	No
12. Would you say your diet is: Good Fair Bad		
13. Do you regularly have breakfast, lunch, and dinner?	Yes	No
14. Do you take vitamins on a daily basis?	Yes	No
15. Is your jaw, head, neck, or back painful now?	Yes	No
16. Have you ever sought advice from a mental health professional for this or any other problem?	Yes	No
17. Do you feel you need treatment for your particular problem?	Yes	No

Headaches		Yes	No
Face Pain		Yes	No
Jaw Pain	Right Left	Yes	No
Neck Aches		Yes	No
Upper Back Aches		Yes	No
Lower Back Aches		Yes	No
Dizziness		Yes	No
Light headedness		Yes	No
Fatigue		Yes	No
Eye Pain	Right Left	Yes	No
Visual Disturbances	Right Left	Yes	No
Post Nasal Drainage		Yes	No
Difficulty Swallowing		Yes	No
Chronic Sore Throat		Yes	No
Difficulty Opening and Closing Mouth		Yes	No
Clicking of Right Jaw Joint		Yes	No
Clicking of Left Jaw Joint		Yes	No
Ear Pain	Right Left	Yes	No
Fullness – Ears and Sinuses	Right Left	Yes	No
Ringing or Buzzing in Ears	Right Left	Yes	No
Pain while eating		Yes	No
Numbness – Arms of Fingers	Right Left	Yes	No

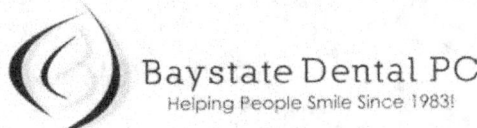

Baystate Dental PC
Helping People Smile Since 1983!

Clinical Exam – Pain on palpation			Maximum Vertical Opening in mm:		
Temporalis	R L		Right Lateral Movement in mm:		
Sternocleidomastoid	R L		Left Lateral Movement in mm:		
Medial Pterygoid	R L		Protrusive Movement in mm:		
Lateral Pterygoid	R L		Click Rt TMJ: Yes No Early Middle Late		
Trapezius	R L		Click Lf TMJ: Yes No Early Middle Late		
Posterior Cervical	R L		Mandibular Movement: Deviation Yes No		
Anterior Cervical	R L		Opening Deviation in mm:		R L
Vertebral Shift	R L		Closing Deviation in mm:		R L
C1	R L		Crepitation:		R L
C2	R L		Pain to joint capsule:		R L N
C3	R L		Pain during clenching:		R L N
C4	R L		Pain on Resting:		R L N
C5	R L		Overbite mm: normal moderately deep substantially deep open		
C6	R L		_____ mm		
C7	R L		Overjet mm: normal moderately deep substantially deep open		
Facial type: Dolichofacial Mesofacial Brachyfacial			_____ mm		
Maxilla: Orthongnathic Retrognathic Prognathic			Crossbite Anterior:		Y N
Mandible: Orthongnathic Retrognathic Prognathic			Crossbite Posteriors:	Y N	RT LF Bilateral
Lower Anterior facial height: long short W.N.L.			Upper Posteriors:	Buccal Lingual	
Gingival display upon smiling:			Freeway Space:	0-3 mm 3-6 mm 6+ mm	
deficient acceptable moderate excessive					
Constricted Max	W.N.L. R L				
Expanded Max	W.N.L. R L				
Facial Symmetry	Symmetric Asymmetric				
Right side:	short neutral long		Left Side:	short neutral long	
Mandible:	Symmetric Asymmetric				
Ramus Portion Long	W.N.L. R L				
Ramus Portion Short	W.N.L. R L				
Body Portion Long	W.N.L. R L				
Body Portion Short	W.N.L. R L				
Lower Occlusal Plain	RT side superior LF side superior Level				
Chewing Patterns	RT only LF only Variable Not aware Uncoordinated Bilat				
Teeth Missing:					
Teeth Present:					
Occlusion RT Molar	I II III		Occlusion RT Cuspid	I II III	
Occlusion LF Molar	I II III		Occlusion LF Cuspid	I II III	
Tongue Thrust Forward	Y N				
Lateral Tongue Thrust	R L N				
Bruxing	Y N				
Clenching	Y N				
Heavy wear facets	Y N				
Forward Head Posture	Y N				
Head Side Bend	R L N				
High Shoulder	R L N				
Low Shoulder	R L N				
Higher Eye	R L N				
Higher Corner of Mouth	R L				
Possible leg length discrepancy	R L				

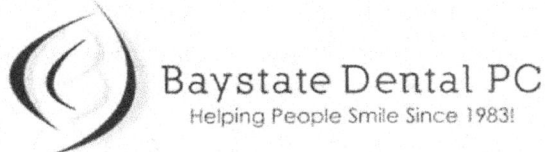

Baystate Dental PC
Helping People Smile Since 1983!

Headache Questionnaire

Name: _____ Date: _____

1. Do you have an idea of what may be causing your headache? (Whiplash, diabetes, high blood pressure, eye strain, etc.)   Yes   No
2. Did this same type of headache ever occur before?   Yes   No
3. Do you have more than one type of headache?   Yes   No
4. Is the headache pain so intense that sometimes it becomes unbearable?   Yes   No
5. Do your headaches occur during stressful tension or nervousness at home, at work, or during social occasions?   Yes   No
6. Does your neck, shoulder muscles, or head junction fell tight and painful during the headache?   Yes   No
7. Is your headache pain dull and steady, like an intense constant pressure? Yes   No
8. Does your headache feel like a tight band around the head?   Yes   No
9. Do you usually have one or more headaches per week?   Yes   No
10. Do your headaches occur during the day?   Yes   No
11. Does your mother, father, or any blood relative have similar headaches?   Yes   No
12. Does exertion (lifting, running, straining, sex) affect your headache?   Yes   No
13. Does nausea and/or vomiting occur before or during your headache?   Yes   No
14. Do you have any changes in vision (flashing lights, sensitivity to light, spots, blurred vision, etc.) before or during your headache?   Yes   No
15. Does your headache usually start on one side of the head?   Yes   No
16. Does your headache throb and pulsate or feel like it is pounding?   Yes   No
17. Do your headaches usually occur during the night or upon awakening?   Yes   No
18. Do your headaches usually occur during weekends and holidays?   Yes   No
19. (Females Only) Is your headache associated with your menstrual period?   Yes   No
20. Do you have watering of the eye on the affected side of the headache?   Yes   No
21. Do alcoholic drinks cause or aggravate your headaches?   Yes   No
22. Does chocolate, cheese, milk, nuts, Chinese food, or any other food cause or worsen your headaches?   Yes   No
23. Do you have any hearing problems – noise, drainage or stuffiness in either ear?   Yes   No
24. Have you noticed any paralysis, muscle weakness, numbness, swallowing problems, or speech changes during your headaches?   Yes   No
25. Do you have any facial pain, aching jaws, stuffiness, or congested sinuses along with your headache?   Yes   No
26. Has it been over eighteen months since you last visited a dentist?   Yes   No
27. Have you had tests for headache? (X-ray, brain scan, injections, etc.)   Yes   No
28. Have you used any previous headache medication? List all medications on the back of this form.   Yes   No

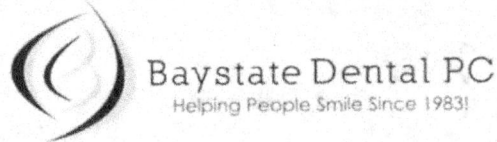

Baystate Dental PC
Helping People Smile Since 1983!

Consent to Decline Neuromuscular Treatment for TMJ

It is the purpose and policy of our practice to always offer our patients treatment options that we consider to be in the best possible interest of the patient. We make every effort to inform our patients of all aspects of recommended treatment and options if there are any. Ultimately, however, the patient decides on their specific treatment and we respect that final decision.

Your initial examination revealed signs and symptoms of jaw dysfunction. It is our opinion that your condition can best be treated by use of neuromuscular principles in enhancing the diagnosis and developing a treatment plan. By your signature hereunder, you acknowledge the following:

a. That we have explained to you that in our considered opinion, a *neuromuscular approach* to your treatment would provide the best possible dental outcome for you in terms of both appearance and function.

b. That we have explained in understandable terms the meaning of neuromuscular based treatment, i.e. that is a method of our establishing the optimal mandibular position for our occlusion (bite) as dictated by first achieving physiological relaxation of the muscles that control your mandible (lower jaw).

c. That we have explained that *traditional dentistry* has <u>not</u> used the neuromuscular mandibular position, but instead has the goal of rebuilding your occlusion (bite) to it present or pre-existing position.

d. While it is possible for the neuromuscular bite and the present or pre-existing bite (called habitual bite) to be the same, it rarely is the same.

You further acknowledge that, having this information clearly explained to you, you have elected to proceed with traditional treatment and to decline treatment based on neuromuscular principles.

Dated: _____

Patient Name: _____
              (Printed Name)

Patient Signature: _____

Doctors' Signature: _____

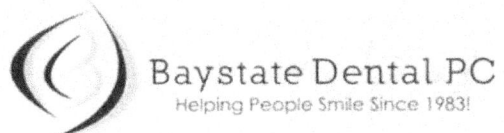

Disclosure Authorization Form

You must follow these instructions when filling out this form.

1.	Sign and date the records release form for only one patient. Complete additional form(s) for each patient.
2.	All signatures must be in black ink and must be original. No copies, facsimiles or stamps are accepted.
3.	Only one signature may appear on a line.
4.	If this form is for a child under the age of 18, a parent or legal guardian must sign for the child.

Permission is given for Baystate Dental PC to disclose □ALL □LIMITED (if limited specify limits in the space below) information in regards to _____ for the following procedures:
(please print name of patient)

_____

_____

_____

to the following individual:

Name:	
Street Address:	
City, State and Zip Code:	
Telephone Number:	( )

I understand that even if I cancel this permission, Baystate Dental PC cannot take back any information that has been released prior to the cancellation request.

Signature of patient:	Date:
Print Name of Patient:	Tel No: ( )
Street Address:	Date of Birth:
City:	State & Zip:

If this form is being filled out by someone who has the legal authority to act on behalf of the patient, (such as the parent of a minor child, an eligibility representative, or a legal guardian), give us the following information:

Signature of person filling out this form:	Date:
Print Name:	Tel No: ( )
Authority of person:	
Please give us a copy of the document that gives you the authority to act on behalf of this patient (driver's license, court order, etc.)	

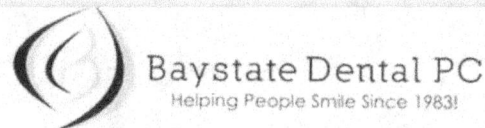

Baystate Dental PC
Helping People Smile Since 1983!

Records Release Form

You must follow these instructions when filling out the records release form.

1.	Sign and date the records release form for only one patient. Complete additional form(s) for each patient.
2.	All signatures must be in black ink and must be original. No copies, facsimiles or stamps are accepted.
3.	Only one signature may appear on a line.
4.	If this form is for a child under the age of 18, a parent or legal guardian must sign for the child.

Permission is given for Baystate Dental PC to release all records, including but not limited to, progress notes, operative notes, laboratory test results, diagnostic tests, and x-rays in regards to
_____ to:
(please print name of patient)

Name Patient, Parent or Legal Guardian:	
Street Address:	
City, State and Zip Code:	
Telephone Number:	( )

I understand that Baystate Dental PC charges a standard copy fee of $_____ for all such release of records and I agree to pay that fee as assessed at the time of this request.

This permission to release all dental records ends six months from the date you sign this release form, unless you cancel permission in writing before the six months has expired.

I understand that even if I cancel this permission, Baystate Dental PC cannot take back any information that has been released prior to the cancellation request.

Signature of patient:	Date:
Print Name of Patient:	Tel No: ( )
Street Address:	Date of Birth:
City:	State & Zip:

If this form is being filled out by someone who has the legal authority to act on behalf of the patient, (such as the parent of a minor child, an eligibility representative, or a legal guardian), give us the following information:

Signature of person filling out this form:	Date:
Print Name:	Tel No: ( )
Authority of person:	
Please give us a copy of the document that gives you the authority to act on behalf of this patient (driver's license, court order, etc.)	

Baystate Dental PC will send you back a copy of this Records Release Form for you to keep for your records. You may also request another copy of this signed Records Release Form at any time by contacting Baystate Dental PC at the following address: Baystate Dental PC, Privacy and Security Office; 1795 Main St, Suite 116, Springfield, MA 01103.

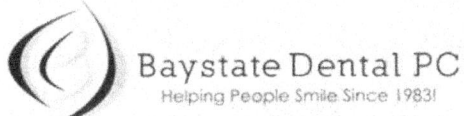

Baystate Dental PC
Helping People Smile Since 1983!

**Administrative Offices at 1795 Main Street
Springfield, Massachusetts 01103**

CONSENT FOR USE AND DISCLOSURE
OF HEALTH INFORMATION

SECTION A: PATIENT GIVING CONSENT

Name: _____

Address: _____

Telephone: _____ Email: _____

Patient#: _____ Social Security#: _____

Section B: TO THE PATIENT – PLEASE READ THE FOLLOWING STATEMENTS CAREFULLY

Purpose of Consent: By signing this form, you will consent to our use and disclosure of your protected health information to carry out treatment, payment activities, and healthcare operations.

Notice of Privacy Practices: You have the right to read our Notice of Privacy Practices before you decide whether to sign this Consent. Our notice provides a description of our treatment, payment activities, and healthcare operations and of the uses and disclosures we may make of your protected health information, and all of other important matters about your protected health information. A copy of our Notice accompanies this Consent. We encourage you to read it carefully before signing this Consent.

We reserve the right to change our privacy practices as described in our Notice of Privacy Practices. If we change our privacy practices, we will issue a revised Notice of Privacy Practices, which will contain the changes. Those changes may apply to any of your protected health information that we maintain.

You may obtain a copy of our Notice of Privacy Practices, including any revisions of our Notice, at any time by contacting:

Contact Person: Scott Massey, Compliance Officer
Telephone: (413) 733-6652 Fax: (413) 439-0563
Email: smassey@baystate-dental.com
Address: Baystate Dental, P.C., 1795 Main Street, Suite 116, Springfield, MA 01103

Right to Revoke: You will have the right to revoke this consent at any time by giving us notice of your revocation submitted to the contact person listed above. Please understand that revocation of this consent will not affect any action we took in reliance on this consent before we received your revocation, and that we may decline to treat you or to continue treating you if you revoke this consent.

SIGNATURE

I, _____, have had full opportunity to read and consider the contents of this Consent form and your Notice of Privacy Practices. I understand that, by signing this Consent form, I am giving my Consent to your use and disclosure of my protected health information to carry out treatment, payment activities and health care operations. I also understand that Baystate Dental PC uses audio and video recorders for training and security purposes.

Signature: _____ Date: _____
If this Consent is signed by a personal representative on behalf of the patient, complete the following:

Personal Representative's Name: _____

Relationship to Patient: _____
YOU ARE ENTITLED TO A COPY OF THIS CONSENT AFTER YOU SIGN IT.

Baystate Dental PC Notice of Privacy Practices

THIS NOTICE DESCRIBES HOW HEALTH INFORMATION ABOUT YOU MAY BE USED AND DISCLOSED AND HOW YOU CAN GET ACCESS TO THIS INFORMATION.

PLEASE REVIEW IT CAREFULLY.

THE PRIVACY OF YOUR HEALTH INFORMATION IS IMPORTANT TO US.

1. OUR LEGAL DUTY

We are required by applicable federal and state law to maintain the privacy of your health information. We are also required to give you this Notice about our privacy practices, our legal duties, and your rights concerning your health information. We must follow the privacy practices that are described in this Notice while it is in effect. This Notice takes effect 09/1/2013, and will remain in effect until we replace it.

We reserve the right to change our privacy practices and the terms of this Notice at any time, provided such changes are permitted by applicable law. We reserve the right to make the changes in our privacy practices and the new terms of our Notice effective for all health information that we maintain, including health information we created or received before we made the changes. Before we make a significant change in our privacy practices, we will change this Notice and make the new Notice available upon request.

You may request a copy of our Notice at any time. For more information about our privacy practices, or for additional copies of this Notice, please contact us using the information at the end of this Notice.

2. USES AND DISCLOSURE OF HEALTH INFORMATION

We use and disclose health information about you for treatment, payment, and healthcare operations. For example:

Treatment: We may use or disclose your health information to a physician or other healthcare provider providing treatment to you.

Payment: We may use and disclose your health information to obtain payment for services we provide to you.

Healthcare Operations: We may use and disclose your health information in connection with our healthcare operations. Healthcare operations include quality assessment and improvement activities, reviewing the competence or qualifications of healthcare professionals, evaluating practitioner and provider performance, conducting training programs, accreditation, certification, licensing or credentialing activities.

Your Authorization: in addition to our use of your health information for treatment, payment or healthcare operations, you may give us written authorization to use your health information or to disclose to anyone for any purpose. If you give us an authorization, you may revoke it in writing at any time. Your revocation will not affect any use or disclosures permitted by your authorization while it was in effect. Unless you give us a written authorization, we cannot use or disclose our health information for any reason except for those described in this Notice.

To Your Family and Friends: We must disclose your health information to you, as described in the Patient Rights section of this Notice. We may disclose your health information to a family member, friend or other person to the extent necessary to help with your healthcare or with payment for your healthcare, but only if you agree that we may do so.

Persons Involved in Care: We may use or disclose health information to notify, or assist in the notification of (including identifying or locating) a family member, your personal representative or another person responsible for your care, of your location, your general condition, or death. If you are present, then prior to use or disclosure of your health information, we will provide you with an opportunity to object to such uses or disclosures. In the event of your incapacity or emergency circumstances, we will disclose health information based on a determination using our professional judgment, disclosing only health information that is directly relevant to the person's involvement in your healthcare.

Marketing Health-Related Services: We will not use your health information for marketing communications without your written authorization.

Abuse or Neglect: We may disclose your health information to appropriate authorities if we reasonably believe that you are a possible victim of abuse, neglect, or domestic violence or the possible victim of other crimes. We may disclose your health information to the extent necessary to avert a serious threat to your health or safety or the heath or safety of others.

National Security: We may disclose to military authorities the health information of Armed Forces personnel under certain circumstances. We may disclose required health information to authorized federal officials for lawful intelligence, counterintelligence, and other national security activities.

Law Enforcement: We may disclose your health information to law enforcement officials as required by law or in compliance with a court order. We may also disclose limited health information to police or law enforcement officials for identification and location purposes and to assist in criminal investigations. We may disclose to correctional institution or law enforcement official having custody of protected health information of inmate or patient under certain circumstances.

Appointment Reminders: We may use or disclose your health information to provide you with appointment reminders (such as email, text message, voicemail messages, postcards, or letters).

3. PATIENT RIGHTS

Access: You have the right to look at or get copies in either printed or electronic format of your health information, with limited exceptions. We will use the format you request unless we cannot practicably do so. You must make a request in writing to obtain access to your health information. You may obtain a form to request access by contacting any of our offices. We will charge you a reasonable cost-based fee for expenses such as copies and staff time of $35.

Disclosure Accounting: You have the right to receive a list of instances in which we or our business associates disclosed your health information for purposes, other than treatment, payment or healthcare operations and certain other activities, for the last 6 years, but not before April 14, 2003. If you request this accounting more than once in a 12-month period, we may charge you a reasonable, cost-based fee for responding to these additional requests.

Restriction: You have the right to request that we place additional restrictions on our use or disclosure of your health information. We are not required to agree to these additional restrictions, but if we do, we will abide by our agreement, except in the event of an emergency.

Alternative Communication: You have the right to request, in writing that we communicate with you about your health information by alternative means or to alternative locations. Your request must specify the alternative means or location, and provide satisfactory explanation how payments will be handled under the alternative means or location you request.

Amendment: You have the right to request that we amend your health information. Your request must be in writing, and it must explain why the information should be amended. We may deny your request under certain circumstances.

Disclosure to Insurance Companies: If you are paying for your treatment in full without using your insurance benefits, you have the right to restrict disclosure of the treatment to your insurance company.

Electronic Notice: If you receive this Notice on our Web site or by electronic mail (e-mail), you are entitled to receive this Notice in written form.

4. QUESTIONS AND COMPLAINTS

If you want more information about our privacy practices, or have questions or concerns, please contact us at any of our offices.

If you are concerned that we may have violated your privacy rights, or if you disagree with a decision we made about access to your health information or in response to a request you made to amend or restrict the use or disclosure of your health information or to have us communicate with you by alternative means or at alternative locations, you may complain to us using the contact information listed at the end of this Notice. You may also submit a written complaint to the U.S. Department of Health and Human Services. We will provide you with the address to file your complaint with the U.S. Department of Health and Human Services upon request.

We support your right to the privacy of your health information. We will not retaliate in any way if you choose to file a complaint with us or with the U.S. Department of Health and Human Services.

Contact: Scott J. Massey
Telephone: 413-733-6651
Fax: 413-439-0563
Address: 1795 Main Street, Suite 116, Springfield, MA 01103

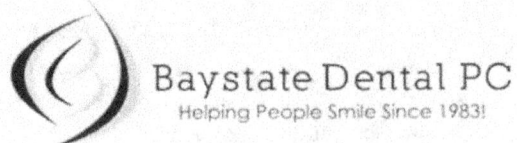

Baystate Dental PC
Helping People Smile Since 1983!

Non-Compliance Form

Baystate Dental PC and it's doctors and employees have explained the risks, benefits, and alternative treatments. They have done their utmost to recommend what they feel will be the most beneficial and successful treatment. After fully understanding the risks, alternatives and benefits, I have elected a dental procedure that the doctor feels will provide less than optimum results and is expected to fail. I have selected this procedure with the full knowledge and the full understanding of my options. As a result of my decision, the following signature will release and forever discharge Baystate Dental PC, its owners, associates, their heirs, employees, agents, officers, directors, assignees, insurers and administrators, collectively from all debts, demands, actions, causes of action, suits, contracts, agreements, damages, costs, expenses, compensation and any and all claims and liabilities of every name and nature including, but not limited to claims for medical expenses, lost earning capacity, disfigurement, pain, suffering, loss of consortium, loss of services, wrongful death, and an such damages past, present or future on account of dental care and treatment.

I understand the above and will not dispute the above claim. Fully understanding the above, I have still agreed to have the procedure preformed based on my wants, needs, and financial considerations and am fully aware that the success of the proposed option is most likely to fail and result in additional expenses and additional care.

Doctor's recommended treatment: _____

Doctor's signature: _____ Date: _____

Patient's choice of treatment: _____

Patient's Name: _____

Patient's signature: _____ Date: _____

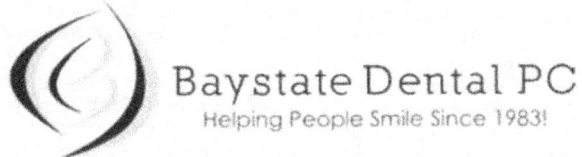

Consent for Non-Covered Services

I have elected to proceed with the following dental treatment and understand that these procedures are not covered services and/or have been denied by my insurance or MassHealth. I understand the fees are my responsibility and they have been fully explained to me.

Procedure	Fee	Date

_____

Patient Name (Please Print)

_____   _____

Signature of Patient (Parent or Legal Guardian)   Date

_____

Doctor Signature